Africana Peoples in China

This book examines the psychosocial experiences of foreign workers from Africa and its diaspora in China, within the context of international socioeconomic forces. By exploring employment-based migration from a psychoanalytic perspective, this volume investigates the utility of adaptive ambivalence and the challenges that migrant workers face around issues of self-development, agency, and identity. Through a careful analysis of interviews with Africana people, the author demonstrates that the capacity to be reflective and resilient alongside having a strong and diversified support network are crucial for the psychological well-being of those living and working in unfamiliar geographical and cultural conditions.

C. Jama Adams is Associate Professor of Psychology and Africana Studies at John Jay College of Criminal Justice/CUNY, USA.

Explorations in Mental Health

Respect-Focused Therapy
Honoring Clients Through the Therapeutic Relationship and Process
Susanne Slay-Westbrook

Depressive Realism
Interdisciplinary Perspectives
Colin Feltham

Families Bereaved by Alcohol or Drugs
Coping and Support
Edited by Christine Valentine

Trans and Sexuality
An Existentially-informed Enquiry with Implications for Counselling Psychology
Christina Richards

Narratives of Loneliness
Multidisciplinary Perspectives from the 21st Century
Edited by Olivia Sagan and Eric D. Miller

Evil Eye, Jinn Possession, and Mental Health Issues
An Islamic Perspective
G. Hussein Rassool

Africana Peoples in China
Psychoanalytic Perspectives on Migration Experiences, Identity, and Precarious Employment
C. Jama Adams

For more information about this series, please visit: www.routledge.com

Africana Peoples in China

Psychoanalytic Perspectives on Migration Experiences, Identity, and Precarious Employment

C. Jama Adams

Routledge
Taylor & Francis Group
NEW YORK AND LONDON

First published 2019
by Routledge
52 Vanderbilt Avenue, New York, NY 10017, USA

and by Routledge
2 Park Square, Milton Park, Abingdon, Oxon, OX14 4RN

First issued in paperback 2020

Routledge is an imprint of the Taylor & Francis Group, an informa business

Library of Congress Cataloguing-in-Publication Data
A catalog record for this book has been requested

ISBN 13: 978-0-367-58502-0 (pbk)
ISBN 13: 978-1-138-34455-6 (hbk)

Typeset in Sabon
by Apex CoVantage, LLC

To my parents and my beloved grandmother

Contents

Acknowledgments

In writing this book, I have benefited from the support of my family, many individuals, and institutions. First, I must thank the many persons in China who took the time to speak with me about their lives and their rich experiences.

Clearly my family's lifelong love and support were crucial in bringing this book to fruition. The experiences and sacrifices of those who were multinational immigrants richly informed my approach to writing this book. Then there were those who gave insightful advice and assistance to a restless youth and to an intermittently befuddled adult. To all of them, I am eternally grateful.

The support of Maureen Denton, Valerie Adams, Edrice Tai, Christine Dwyer and Robert Grossmark was above and beyond the call of duty. I express my heartfelt thanks to them.

I thank Marissa Dennis, Eve Golden, and Eliza Mason for their insightful comments on many drafts of chapters for this book and Kristopher Spring for his eagle-eye editing.

I very much appreciate Yoon Jung Park of the China Africa/Africa China Network encouragement, recommending me for conference panels and presentations, and her sharing of contacts.

John Jay College of Criminal Justice through its Office of Academic Research was generous in its funding my attendance at various conferences and in paying for editing services.

The process of transforming a scattered manuscript into a coherent work was superbly facilitated by Kate Hawes, Matt Friberg, Katherine Tsamparlis, and the staff of Routledge Publishing.

1 Introduction

Africana peoples have been restless migrants from the dawn of Homo sapiens and embody human curiosity. As part of different waves of globalization, they have suffered being commodified and dehumanized. In addition, many have found themselves embedded in oppressive structures that have limited their access to the resources necessary to develop the capabilities that in turn make agency possible. The latest iteration of globalization has opened up considerable opportunities for wealth generation and self-discovery, especially in China. As a result Africana persons from Africa and its vast diaspora are going to China, among other places. There they must adaptively manage the ambivalence manifested as excitement at the opportunities for skilled employment and wealth creation, alongside limits on spirituality, intimacy, and community building.

Initial Attraction to the Topic of Africana People in China

"Wherever he goes the Negro remains a Negro," wrote Frantz Fanon (1967, p. 173) in *Black Skin, White Masks*, and that invariably means a denial of a common humanity, restrictions on access to resources, and limits on agency and self-growth. I thought about Fanon's assertion and my own intellectual curiosity in the humid summer heat of Shanghai in 2010 as I explored the city and visited the World Expo. I had gone to Shanghai not only as a tourist, but also as a psychologist and a scholar of the social sciences with an interest in difference, commonalities, and macro forces that influence how people love and work. I wondered whether Fanon's dispiriting trajectory was also evident in the experiences of Africana persons in China more than 40 years after he wrote about it. By Africana, I mean persons from continental Africa or the African diaspora.

This is all framed by the awareness of being embedded in a globalized system of a long-standing and protean capitalism that commodifies all that it touches. At the same time, it also provides life-changing opportunities for the creative person who is disciplined, perceptive, and embedded in supportive and well-endowed networks. One example of this is that of my mother, who journeyed to Liverpool in England, the former major European slave port, in response to a shortage of labor in the health care services in the late 1940s. She was one of many relatives who traveled north also in search of wealth and self-development. There was also a great aunt who worked in the United States during the depression and my Somali father who was a sailor and part of a wide-flung and tragedy-tinged diaspora.

To look at Liverpool, where I was born, is to see remnants of the profits derived from buying and selling Africana bodies. These market forces continue to influence the movements of hundreds of millions of people, including those of Africana heritage in China and elsewhere. To look at my extended families is to locate relatives on every major land mass except Australia. Such is the power of both human curiosity and globalized capital.

As part of my research, over the course of the following few years, the inquiry that began on this trip developed into a focused interest, and I committed to write about it. I therefore visited a few locales in southeast China where the bulk of Africana persons were located, and I thought that the commercial district in Guangzhou captured in some ways the strivings of the Africana workers within the context of a globalized business setting. The frenetic commercial district in Guangzhou where many African traders are located was a seemingly familiar scene located in a Chinese place. From afar, I observed on the street the usual and purposeful movement of multitasking businesspeople; they were mostly fairly tall and dark skinned, and were often robed African men who were on cell phones or in multilingual clusters having intense conversations. Interspersed was the occasional African businesswoman clad in ethnic dress and serious of countenance. One imagined that they were focused on business transactions or related administrative challenges. On closer inspection, however, what was different about this space in China was partially revealed: Here there was an abundance of dark-skinned persons, probably of African heritage, who could be found engaging with Chinese persons in varying ways. Some worked as vigilant suppliers of goods or intermediaries, others were ever-hurrying drivers or delivery persons, and still others deployed different kinds of agency, including the responsibility for negotiating with the municipal authorities with regard to the implementation of administrative policies that support the needs of foreign businesspersons. I also heard about low-keyed but increasing advocacy efforts by Africana groups in southern China who were, and still are, fighting for fair treatment by law enforcement and immigration authorities

As I paused on the corner on my way to interview a subject one afternoon, in my capacity as an Africana scholar trained in clinical psychology but with broader sociocultural interests, I knew I was in China, but I couldn't help but feel like this particular area of Guangzhou was a very

Africana-informed China, compared to say the commercial sector of Shanghai or the art enclave in Beijing, places with which I was somewhat familiar. I opened my ears and listened: I hardly heard Chinese or the imperial languages, French and English. Instead, African indigenous languages were dominant among African traders, and the Chinese businesspersons spoke their local Chinese variants. This meant that African buyers and Chinese businesspeople often did not share a substantive common language. Instead, interactions between these two groups took place in what Bodomo (2012) has termed "calculator communication" (p. 43), referring to the tangible brew of diaspora linguistics, profit motives, and the use of the calculator as a medium of communication. I of course couldn't understand the verbal give-and-take, but realized that this compromise—the back-and-forth passing of the calculator until an agreement in the purchase price was made—was a simple but clear manifestation of the growth of south-to-south interactions and market-driven transactions.

I observed these business practices for a while—standing off to the side, observing traders sitting and waiting with their goods for transportation to arrive and seeing the odd African and Chinese couple going by. Yet the more I observed, the less comfortable I felt trying to facilely categorize the multiplicity of sounds and images. I saw both Chinese and Africana persons weaving in and out of traffic while others were loading vehicles, blithely ignoring the disruptions they were causing to the flow of vehicles. This casual disregard for traffic laws was very much Chinese, but also very much West African. The etiquette of walking was New York-like—move quickly and try not to touch anyone—but with this being China, there was less personal space. There was also evident the cultural infrastructure of an Africana community: mosques, African-themed restaurants, nightclubs, and service businesses offering food, entertainment, spiritual sustenance or various purchasing, shipping, and brokerage services.

This awareness of commonalties between me and these Africana workers in terms of the assertion of agency, combined with an exploration of human responses to pervasive market forces, sometimes slavishly, and at other times adroitly, constitutes the major foci of this work.

Affinities and Cautions

I am definitely what Conway (2007) and Said (1993) among others mean when they refer to those of us who live in "in-between-ness." This is a state of *otherness* that offers unique perspectives alongside a sense of never quite fitting in and never quite being fully recognized, accompanied by eddies of melancholia and waves of joy. As a result of my own peripatetic childhood, I assumed a certain affinity with these Africana persons in China, who were living away from home and yet had established a new one, however transient. I also knew that there were profound differences between us, as the complexities of one's cultural heritage always involve a concomitant struggle over the ideas of categorization itself, taking into consideration both similarities and dissimilarities. This meant that for as many connections as I could draw between my own experiences and those of the Africana workers in China, we were in some other ways worlds apart.

They came to China from Africa and from its diverse diaspora for a range of reasons: on scholarships to study at Chinese universities, as traders shuttling between southern China and mostly West Africa, as recruited executives working for Chinese and Western corporations, and as teachers of English scattered across the country. It became quickly evident to me that complex cultural and psychological contingencies were influencing the presence of these folks in China and that I might be able to bring a multidisciplinary perspective to bear on what I was observing. They were in a culture that was quite different than any that most Africana people, including me, had ever experienced. At the same time, I had often wondered about the commonality of oppression that Black folks experienced wherever they resided. Would China be different? Would the capitalist and nationalist-driven demand for creative workers trump China's antipathy to foreigners? How would the ascendant market ethos inform relations between the variegated self-interests of the Chinese and their Africana sojourners? Would there be places within which otherness could be explored without the necessity to denigrate, subordinate, or marginalize?

As I researched further, I saw that there are clusters of Africana persons in China that share weak commonalities. In addition to the mostly traders in Guangzhou, there is also a distinct and diverse cohort of Africana persons in Shanghai, although they do not, as a whole, share strong identifications or links with the Guangzhou trading community. Its members are widely dispersed, rely heavily on the internet as a way of communicating, and maintain some semblance of community. Such persons are academically credentialed individuals, some of whom work for Western and others for Chinese corporations. Other Africana workers are employed as English teachers and can be found in diverse locales throughout China. The same can be said for foreign students, who, of all the Africana groups in China, tend to be the most fluent and literate in Chinese. The majority are required to take a 10-month immersion course in Chinese prior to starting their formal studies.

Persons of Africana heritage have been living in various parts of China, but especially in southern China, Beijing, and Shanghai, in significant numbers, since the late 1990s. This upsurge was, in part, a response to increased economic opportunities in China (Adams, 2015; Bodomo, 2012). It is difficult to get an accurate estimate of how many Africana persons reside in China, given the sporadic availability and questionable accuracy of any number given by official and other sources (Castillo, 2016; Haugen, 2015). Estimates are as low as 20,000 and as high as 100,000 in some parts (Bodomo, 2012; Castillo, 2016). These Africana persons working in China are best referred to as "foreign workers" since, under Chinese law, it is extremely difficult for foreigners to be granted permanent resident status or to become naturalized Chinese citizens. Until quite recently, China had no established pathway to permanent residency or citizenship for foreigners, nor until recently did there appear to be a central government administrative structure for immigration matters. This was consistent with the larger assumption that foreigners are not expected to reside permanently in China together with the apparent general desire that they not do so. This policy is beginning to change as China becomes more integrated, albeit selectively, into the global community and China's need for diverse sources of talent and skills (China Law & Practice, 2012).

China nevertheless conveys that foreign workers' stay in China will be temporary no matter how long they live there and, in turn, many Africana people seem to accept this stance. The nationalistic hue of this attitude toward foreign workers, while very evident in China and perhaps more so in Japan (Oishi, 2012), is not unique to those nations. Such an approach was long a feature of post-World War II German policies toward its Turkish "guest workers" (Munz & Ulrich, 2004) and is also evident in British immigration policies (Spencer, 1997). Workers are needed, but migrants are shunned. Evident here is the subordination of the workers' non-economic interests to those of the market.

Most foreigners in China are granted a 1-year visa that must be renewed annually at a Chinese embassy or consulate outside of mainland China. Former subjects of my study have informed me that in 2016, the supporting documentation demands increased considerably. The assumption is that they are temporary residents, and yet some report up to 25 years of annual renewals of their "temporary" status. This annual official reinforcement of the foreigner's outsider status can discourage any substantive material or emotional investment in China, given that their application for renewal can be refused at any point in time.

Africana workers in China are the beneficiaries of declining costs of information, transportation, and communication. Two consequences of these changes are an increase in south-to-south trade and an increase in demand for skilled workers. These changes present opportunities for the Africana workers to nurture a sense of competency and autonomy that was difficult to achieve in their respective home countries or communities, given their structural limitations. There are, however, also risks to the self, generated by those same forces. The individual must increasingly be aware of the challenges that the dominant neoliberal market ethos presents to living a life that is not limited to selling skills, engaging in thoughtless consumption, and attenuated ties and obligations to community. The abundance of available information also includes inaccuracies and misrepresentations that make the Africana person vulnerable to exploitation. I heard stories of internet-based scams for nonexistent jobs and struggles to ensure that goods were manufactured to the agreed specifications and using the agreed-upon quality of materials. There were endless stories of contracts that were not honored and blatant racism. I will offer some detailed examples of these types of experiences in the chapters that follow.

Behind the material risks, of which there are many, lie still other risks such as that of existential homelessness. This can be the unfortunate outcome where, despite the apparent ease with which one can live, there exists a seemingly bearable lightness of being and yet a longing to be grounded. Akin to the characters in Milan Kundera's (2005) book, *The Unbearable Lightness of Being*, Africana individuals living and working in China risk being uncommitted to a degree that makes the individual who is overly attracted to being unfettered vulnerable to being alienated.

Again, the seductions of the market, often attractive to long-thwarted desires, if not well managed, make it difficult for the Africana person not to switch one set of self-constraints for another. They have left places of too many limits on curiosity, self-awareness, and wealth accumulation. The challenge is that in China, even as they exploit the opportunity to develop market-oriented capabilities, they must resist the distraction of mindless consumption and must also be attentive to social constraints on rights, religiosity, and community organizing. Wherever they are, they will be constrained and must come to terms with that as they pursue opportunities.

Psychological Challenges

The Market and the Self

The market facilitates, constrains, and distorts the migrant's developmental aspirations (de Haas, 2010), including those of Africana persons in China. Market forces are a major influencing factor in migrants' decision to leave their home countries and as to why they are in China; these market forces, often unacknowledged, act to facilitate some forms of self-development, while inhibiting others. Through globalization, the market offers infinite models of ways of being, of tactics to enhance agency and therefore mobility, but in some of its more seductive and prominent iterations, these models privilege a particular set of benchmarks, often narcissistic, consumerist, and cognitively oriented, for assessing progress in self-development. Given its selective nature, the market can appear to marginalize being reflective and other qualities for which there is no apparent desire or those which cannot be easily commodified. The market also often exacerbates the tension between the nurturance of community and the pursuit of self-interests. In China, material self-interests are often unwittingly reinforced by state policies that are wary of group efforts to organize community and the advocacy efforts that such resulting networks often give rise to.

Issues such as ethical relating and the demand for state-sponsored protection of basic rights, meet with indifference or, as is sometimes the case in China, hostility. What is increasingly apparent in an age of mature capitalism is a preference for the cultivation of the primordial and intellectual aspects of self in the service of consumption.

Market values in China, among other places, are increasingly very influential in defining some of the goals of self-development (Kipnis, 2007). Recognition, a central goal of the individual, is often defined in terms of technical intellectual skills, creativity, and material wealth. Such recognition is selective as it does not acknowledge all aspects of the individual, but only those that are in the service of the production and consumption of what is in demand in the financially driven marketplace (Crouch, 2016). Less recognized, and often resisted, are appeals for human rights, spirituality, protection, and accountability. This is especially the case for Africana workers in China, where there exists the opportunity to develop a sense of agency and efficacy with regard to the acquisition and deployment of intellectual skills. It also presents opportunities to acquire financial surpluses and material goods to a degree difficult to attain in the home country.

The Sense of Being Other and In-Between-Ness

There are, however, substantive limits on recognition and inclusion, and the building of community; actions that are crucial for healthy well-being. Africana workers are perceived as foreigners and are unlikely to be granted permanent residence status in China, no matter how long they reside. China is therefore a place of much uncertainty that offers opportunity for the perceptive and the skilled, but also the pain of the arbitrariness that periodically comes from being in an authoritarian system in flux. The state often seems wary of the foreigner as a bearer of values that are a threat to the status quo with regard to recognition, inclusion, and the rights demands arising from that.

This sense of partial recognition and exclusion is psychologically costly and an inherent feature of being an Africana person in China, with both its wariness of foreigners and its objectifying market ethos. It heightens a sense of ambivalence that originated in the home country, a sense of being always, to some degree, *other*, given being thwarted at home in attempts at self-development, especially with regard to intellectual pursuits and the generation of wealth. A related psychological challenge especially relevant to the Africana person and to the foreigner is that of recognition and identity. This is evident in the marginalization of their histories of struggle and the wish to be acknowledged as human beings and as citizens. Such struggles can be all too familiar to Africana persons who are from home countries that were former colonies or who were at one time embedded in embattled and devalued diasporic communities that are under the yoke of politically illiberal and economically neoliberal regimes.

For Africana people, there is always a sense, whether at home or abroad of not quite belonging. This subjective sense of *otherness* is muted in the home country but is explicitly felt in the host country resulting in such individuals often experiencing the psychological state of in-between-ness, not quite belonging regardless of where they reside (Conway, 2007; Said, 1993).

In China, there is not much state-sponsored attention to addressing the emotional concerns of the individual (Kleinman et al., 2011). What one observes is the privatization of affect: Loss, loneliness, the sense of exclusion, the ignoring of intergenerational pain, and the hidden transcripts of the subjective must be managed outside of the official discourses that inform policy (Benduce, 2008). This sense of an underlay of psychic incompleteness and stymied potential arising from complimentary and unethical constraints on self-development is experienced at both the structural and interpersonal level. The Africana person is often embedded in situations both at home and in the host country where the state offers low levels of nurturance and protection and limits ethical appeals for rights, services, and inclusion.

Adaptive Ambivalence

The challenge then for Africana people abroad is to develop adaptive ways of managing their ambivalence toward both home and host countries. This speaks to accepting that being perceived as other and therefore different is an inherent feature of the modern condition, resulting in an ontological questioning of the meaning of home and of identity (Strenger, 2013; Tsolidis, 2014). One consequence is that individuals must find adaptive ways of managing this sense of existential unease, the not quite belonging, the risks of being un-moored, and a lightness of being. They are at times grudgingly granted partial recognitions and can construct places within which to engage in healthy self-making.

Traditional Psychological Models of Migration

The traditional perspective with regard to the exploration of the psychological features of immigrants has been to focus on them as engaging in a trauma-producing event as they relinquishes precious ties to the home country and over time adapt to the host country that becomes the new home (Grinberg & Grinberg, 1982). The assumption appeared to be that the losses were irreversible and that the host country was benign and accepting. Traditional perspectives reflected the reality that while there were potent fantasies of return to the home country (Akhtar, 1995), they were unrealizable. This included the possibility of sojourning, given the paucity of the psychological and socioeconomic factors that could make that possible (Selvon, 1989). Given that context, it made sense to view the idea of migration as traumatic with little thought that for many, the experience could be a joyful act of exploration and self-development. Little attention was paid as to how market forces impacted self-improvement beyond acknowledging the pursuit of skills and material resources.

The idea of the foreign worker, while not new, did not in the post-World War II era encompass an awareness of the sharp objectification of such a worker. Neither was there much focus on the actions of a state apparatus, guided by both nationalistic and increasingly by market norms. Here the intent is the exploitation of foreign workers and at the same time limiting or excluding such persons' access to the rights and benefits of the national community.

Core Perspectives on the Africana Workers in China

Structure and Agency

I will argue throughout this book that the Africana subjectivities being examined can be best explored at the intersection of two narratives: one that considers the broader structural forces that interact with the individual's subjectivities and another that encompasses the particular, quotidian actions that both facilitate and constrain certain kinds of individual agency. The outcome would be the degree to which individuals can adaptively manage the ambivalence generated by their state of in-between-ness. It would seem that the experiences of Africana workers in China is but one manifestation of a growing phenomenon of foreign individuals struggling for recognition by host countries and destined not to have it completely granted. Given that, one observes the evolution of a way of managing the self that I term *adaptive ambivalence*. If such a state is well managed, it functions as a buffer against the more costly risks of managing the dispiriting aspects of the ever restless modernity in which the individual is embedded.

The structural narrative, as outlined above, must by necessity include the political, economic, social, and cultural paradigms present in transnational forces, the migrants' home country, and in China, which is to say a multi-determined and transnational narrative. In the context of the host country, this would speak to the opportunities that are available to the Africana person to develop intellectually as well as the availability of meaningful and well-paying work. That in turn would possibly create places within which to work on other aspects of self-development.

Such a perspective would also include the cultural narratives around transnational movements, immigration, ethics, and the nurturance of community. Less evident but still present would be approaches to embracing diverse and not necessarily always comfortable ways of being different. This is perhaps most important for our current considerations—it includes pipelines for exporting the "restless *Other*," the one who does not quite fit in, and so it includes as well ways of managing complex ideas around longing and disenchantment with home, wherever that may be.

Under-thematization of Migrants' Subjectivities

There is very little literature on the subjectivities of Africana foreign workers in China; this is reflective of the fact that this is a population of relatively recent origin. It is also an indication of a particular bias in the migration literature that, until recently, has tended to focus on transnational workers as economic actors with relatively little attention to other aspects of their aspirations (de Haas, 2010). Related to this is a tendency to limit attention to immigrant subjectivities to that of loss and mourning with little mention of adaptation, hybridity, ambition, hope, increased agency, or ambivalence. There is also little attention to the interplay between subjective factors and the structures within which the individual is, by necessity, embedded. Finally, also contributing to this lack is the long-standing focus on migration from the south to north, or east to west, with little attention being paid to the long-existing and growing south-to-south commerce and migration patterns.

The exploration of the subjectivities of transnational workers and immigrants is therefore an under-thematized subject in the research literature, a lack that this book will attempt, at least partially, to correct. This lack becomes more significant when coupled with the equally under-thematized issue of the subjectivities of Africana persons. The focus of this book will therefore be on the adaptive management of the ambivalence that is an inherent feature of being an Africana worker in China. The possibilities for self-development are both facilitated and constrained by the cultural contexts within which the individual is embedded. So I will seek to understand the ways in which structure in some of its permutations both constrains and makes possible certain experiences of personal development (Chun, 2009). Finally, where this book also makes a unique contribution is in the use of a psychodynamic framework to attempt to understand the subjective experience of migration more generally, and Africana migrant experiences in China more specifically. By stating that I use a psychodynamic framework, I mean looking at how elation, sense of efficacy, conflict, melancholy, frustrations, and anxieties, among other subjective states, are managed—not necessarily consciously—by the Africana individual who is living in China.

It should also be noted that, as is the case with all ethnographic and theoretical work, embedded in the various narrative strands will be both a critique of the extant literature and thoughts on how such literature could be reimagined. This is not to say that I have all the answers, nor is it to say that extant literature has not contributed much to the field. On the contrary, my point of view will be this one: that an attempt to theorize Africana subjectivities in a Chinese context allows us to speak to possibility, constraints, and the management—both my own and theoretical—of the resulting tensions. It is in the tangled form of this conundrum, I believe, that we can find the richest possibilities for understanding.

Ambivalence Among Africana Persons in China

In interacting with Africana merchants in Guangzhou and with other Africana professionals in Shanghai, I sensed that many experienced a degree of ambivalence about their experiences in China. Many were pleased with their respective achievements in China; they had made money, some had purchased comfortable homes, and in some cases the Africana men had married Chinese women. In my six field trips to China between 2012 and 2014, I consistently heard stories with similar themes of personal growth, along with a sense of increased autonomy and less constriction around work life than these Africana foreign workers had experienced in their respective home countries. At the same time, though, these workers had faced and continued to face considerable difficulties. Many of the people I talked to were not overly enthused about being in China given the obstacles they faced—problems that included such mundane but essential tasks such as the annual visa renewal. They also had to cope with experiences of systemic inequalities including corruption and racial discrimination, not to mention the infrequent but sometimes jarring reminders that they were both Black and foreign. So for example, in Guangzhou, it is not unusual for Africana workers to be caught up in immigration sweeps aimed at apprehending undocumented persons of Africana heritage. Vigilance is the twin sibling of hustling in this ancient trading center.

Many of these Africana foreign workers also faced another source of frustration: their ongoing concerns about being exploited given their unfamiliarity with Chinese business and administrative practices, which together comprised a system that was often experienced as unethical, corrupt, objectifying, and arbitrary. Many Africana merchants, for example, discovered painfully that the standard West African practice of bargaining to get a lower price for the same quality product was not the norm in China. Instead, they reported that a Chinese supplier, with whom they may not be able to communicate proficiently in Chinese, might lower his price, but he would also lower the quality of the goods supplied. Many of the Africana workers in China, regardless of status, often felt that they were objectified by the Chinese, who they felt were only interested in their technical expertise and in their financial resources. Among the traders in Guangzhou, there was some bitterness that the administrative authorities did not acknowledge their contributions to Chinese economic growth, while among the technocrats working mostly in Shanghai, there was the sense that they too were objectified with a focus on their skills but little interest in other aspects of their being.

Such apparent Chinese behaviors might be attributed, in part, to the migrants' collective lack of Chinese language skills and also to the authorities' ambivalence regarding the presence of these Africana persons, although that is, of course, not the whole story. Despite these substantial challenges, among many Africana workers, there was a sense of having created a psychological place that enabled them to fruitfully work the tension between the attractions and disappointments of both home and China, which gave rise to a stance that I refer to as adaptive ambivalence. They sought to understand and hold in tension both the gratifying and the constraining aspects of both the home and the host country with the goal of actively managing their ambivalence. They sought to come to terms with the awareness that neither place was idyllic, but at the same time, each offered some psychic gratification in relation to its constraints.

Africana Subjectivities

Adding to the complexity of the external structure and the constraints of the social space was the following question: What were some of the features of the subjectivities of these busy vanguard foreign workers? I use the term *workers* deliberately as many have no intention of remaining in China, and, as I have mentioned, China's immigration policies make it very difficult to gain permanency status. The Africana workers in China whom I met were a long way from home—a place about which, in many ways, they also felt ambivalent and somewhat ill-at-ease, as they did not feel that there was adequate support there for their local attempts at personal development. Now they were in a place that, again, while supportive of certain attempts at self-development, was not a full-fledged support system; they did not entertain a vision of China as a substantive second home given their experience of wariness on the part of many Chinese people and institutions toward them. In addition, many have been stymied and perturbed by the structural constraints that impede attempts at self-growth in the areas of intimacy, religion, and rights advocacy. At the same time, a paradox emerged: Many Africana persons reported a sense of growth in areas such as autonomy, tolerance, and worldliness, and a degree and quality of thoughtfulness in relation to themselves that had not been evident at home. This means that while there was a sense of being *other* at home, there was a sense of growth in China that existed alongside the experience of being *other* there as well.

While we know some of the reasons that people leave their homelands in search of a better future—one that is both economically and personally fulfilling—it is my contention that we don't yet know enough about their internal motivations and the subjective experiences of migration and work that are facilitated through such transnational movements. These workers' understanding of themselves, their fantasies, the push for agency, the sources of emotional nurturance, the inevitable compromises, and their anxieties remain largely unknown. It is my hope that this book can shed some new light on this particular subject matter through theoretical exploration and from the stories told to me by Africana migrants living in China.

Researcher Subjectivities

My approach to this project presents me with certain risks, such as the importance of being aware of and managing my projections. It would be easy and familiar to measure progress for the Africana person in China as solely manifested by some state of mind that transcends skill-oriented knowledge and the acquisition of material goods. Such a tendency would be fueled—either consciously or unconsciously—by my own experiences of never having had to be overly preoccupied with obstacles to the acquisition of formal academic qualifications or material resources. Given my sufficiently adequate support network, it was always expected that I would perform well in the academic realm. There was rarely any mention of the structural limits on developing talent or of the fact that so many of my own family members felt the need to migrate given the structural inadequacies of home. Issues of a sense of loss and longing were never mentioned, perhaps because leaving was such a normal developmental milestone for so many—an all-too-familiar rite of passage to which I and countless others were subjected.

Many people coming from modest economic means may justly and proudly assess themselves as being successful if they can attain reasonable levels of formal education, skill development, material surplus, and stability, as well as the modest increase in status that might come with such achievements. At the same time, even as they fiercely strive for cognitive enrichment and material security, there is often a sense that the importance of emotional and spiritual well-being ought not to be sacrificed in pursuit of the economic and the material. For some there is a painful awareness of being unfulfilled, lacking the feeling of being recognized and respected, and experiencing a need to contribute to and feel embedded in a caring and protective community.

My orientation impacts the type of story I am able to tell. Part of my role as researcher involves carefully managing different perspectives. This includes theories, prominent in certain Western and Chinese precincts, that hold that those who do not excel by orienting toward a neoliberal market ethos, expressed in part through the outward manifestation of exceptional individuality and control of an abundance of resources, have somehow failed. This is a position that researchers must question. This is especially the case when deploying psychoanalytic perspectives that often seem indifferent to the socioeconomic factors that, when well managed, facilitate personal development but can often impinge on and make shallow the quality of that pursuit. The fulfillment of basic needs, a more challenging task in these neoliberal inflected times, will often give rise to the contemplation and pursuit of more elusive but deeply gratifying and enduring subjectivities. The challenge is to avoid the tendency to perceive the pursuit of the material and the enchanted as implacable and unattainable binaries.

Subjects and Methodology

In this study, I focus on Africana persons residing in China who share a weak commonality in being of African heritage, identifying with a connection to Africa. In its most common iteration, there is from the perspective of family, either a direct or ancestral connection to Africa. Another use of Africana as a common signifier is its interpretation and ascription by the Chinese. Individuals in China with dark skin are often perceived as being "Black" or "African" although they may not necessarily define themselves as such.

The data cited is based on fieldwork that I did in Shanghai and Guangzhou from 2010 to 2013, and the research was approved by John Jay College's Institutional Review Board. Subjects were recruited through word of mouth and referrals from trusted leaders of community organizations in Shanghai and Guangzhou. I strived to interview a wide range of subjects so as to elicit a diverse range of experiences and to avoid an overrepresentation of any one of the work groups described below. So, for example, it is relatively easy to interview traders, students, and English teachers. It is harder to locate and interview artists, affluent entrepreneurs, and senior executives.

The subject pool consists of 41 individuals of Africana heritage from Africa, the Caribbean, Europe, and North America from home countries in 17 different nation states. Twenty-three subjects were male, and 18 were female. Ages ranged from 21 to 61 with most subjects being in their mid-30s. Most had resided in China for less than 5 years, while a few had lived there for over 15 years. The overwhelming majority did not consider themselves fluent in Chinese, but most could negotiate simple social and business transactions in Chinese. Most of the students who had been studying in Chinese universities for more than 2 years were literate and orally proficient in Chinese.

Subjects belonged to one of the following work groups: students, traders, entrepreneurs, English teachers, consultants, and technocrats. Managers working in corporate offices resided in Shanghai, while most of the traders resided in Guangzhou. While I did not inquire directly about their immigration status in China, most immigrants described frequent trips abroad, which would suggest that they had valid visas. Two immigrant men had Chinese wives and bicultural children born in China, but there were no Africana women in the subject pool who had Chinese husbands or partners. I also drew on data collected by Haugen and Diederich (2016a, 2016b, 2016c, 2016d, 2016e, 2016f) on low-functioning Gambians in China and on internet sites dealing with various aspects of being Africana in China.

The sample described here is skewed toward university-educated subjects who have valid immigration documents and earn good salaries. They tend to be workers with formal training who are actively recruited and hired in a talent area lacking in China such as English language proficiency, creative work, or technological prowess, and so they are usually well paid and are assisted in maintaining their legal residency status. Most of the traders in the sample, but not all, were small businessmen in a reportedly ethically challenged and cutthroat business milieu with low profit margins and low levels of social trust between themselves and the Chinese and sometimes with other Africana workers. Many relied heavily on unscrupulous brokers to obtain and renew their visas and had to be vigilant against arbitrary arrest by the police or the immigration authorities (Haugen, 2012).Data was collected using a structured protocol with all subjects being interviewed in English. Transcripts were analyzed based on selected themes arising from psychoanalytic and sociological perspectives on agency, structure, self, and identity. Also explored were themes emerging from the psychologically attuned literature on the experience of being an immigrant. Family structures and other network supports were carefully examined in the context of factors that influence and support migration.

Some methodological limitations are evident in this work. The first is that this is a small, unrepresentative sample of Africana persons in China and does not include subjects from a sizable and long-standing presence of Africana persons in Macau since the seventeenth century (Morais, 2009). Another cautionary point is the transient nature of the Africana population in China. Students and executives are in China for a limited period of time, and most leave with no plans to return while many traders engage in "shuttle migration," moving between their home countries and China on a regular basis (Bodomo, 2012). One therefore must speak tentatively about an Africana community in China given the high degree of movement into and out of China. As an alternative, many persons are embedded in networks where the focus is on information sharing but there is a lack of a strong affective component.

Also missing is any direct substantive sense of how the Chinese perceive the Africana persons in their midst. My Chinese language limitations and that of most of the subjects made it difficult to access that perspective. I was able to draw on some internet sources and research papers providing they were in English.

Aim of the Book

The aim of the book is to convey a sense of the experience of foreign workers in a host country with a focus of Africana people in China. The aim is to highlight the pleasures and challenges subjectively experienced, with an emphasis on the interplay between individuals' sense of agency and the structures in which they are embedded. I begin with an exploration of adaptive ambivalence: the interplay of initiative and compromise alongside the emotional vicissitudes that arise. Then I lay out the features of modernity and the ways in which it facilitates the current role of capitalism and globalization. Carefully explored are the ways in which dominant ways of thinking such as capitalism influence individuals' dreams, aspirations, and compromises. The tension in China is between features of modernity that can facilitate much needed economic growth and service provision, and at the same time, an antipathy toward modernity-driven issues such as cultural diversity and innovation in the political sector. The following chapters focus on the history of African persons in China and their contemporary experiences within the context of self-making. I end with some speculative thoughts about the future of Blackness in China.

References

Adams, C. J. (2015). Structure and agency: Africana immigrants in China. *Journal of Pan African Studies*, *7*(10), 85–108.

Akhtar, S. (1995). A third individuation: Immigration, identity and the psychoanalytic process. *Journal of the American Psychoanalytic Association*, *43*(4), 1051–1084.

Benduce, R. (2008). Undocumented bodies, buried identities: Refugees, sans papiers, harraga-when things fall apart. *Social Science Information*, *47*(4), 505–527.

Bodomo, A. (2012). *Africans in China*. Amherst, NY: Cambria Press.

Castillo, R. (2016). How many Africans are in Guangzhou? Retrieved from https://africansinchina.net/how-many-africans-are-there-in-guangzhou/

China Law & Practice. (2012). China's new immigration law explained. Retrieved from www.chinalawandpractice.com/Article/3060403/Channel/9931/Chinas-new-Immigration-Law-explained.html

Chun, A. (2009). On the geopolitics of identity. *Anthropological Theory*, *9*(3), 331–349.

Conway, D. (2007). Caribbean transnational migration behavior: Reconceptualizing its "strategic flexibility." *Population, Space and Place*, *13*, 415–431.

Crouch, C. (2016). *The knowledge corrupters: Hidden consequences of the financial takeover of public life*. Cambridge, UK: Polity Press.
de Haas, H. (2010). Migration transitions: A theoretical and empirical inquiry into the developmental drivers of international migration (DEMIG working paper, University of Oxford: International Migration Institute).
Fanon, F. (1967). *Black skin, white masks*. New York, NY: Grove Press.
Grinberg, L., & Grinberg, R. (1982). *Psychoanalytic perspectives on migration and exile*. New Haven, CT: Yale University Press.
Haugen, H. (2012). Nigerians in China: A second state of immobility. *International Migration*, *50*(2), 65–80.
Haugen, H. (2015). Destination China: The country adjusts to its new migration reality. Retrieved from http://migrationpolicy.org/article/destination-china-country-adjusts-its-new-migration-reality
Haugen, H., & Diederich, M. (2016a). Decision to leave home. Retrieved from https://uturnasia.com/2016/01/26/test/
Haugen, H., & Diederich, M. (2016b). From the Gambia to China. Retrieved from https://uturnasia.com/2016/01/25/test11/
Haugen, H., & Diederich, M. (2016c). Life in China. Retrieved from https://uturnasia.com/2016/01/24/test-1/
Haugen, H., & Diederich, M. (2016d). Getting out of China. Retrieved from https://uturnasia.com/2016/01/23/18/
Haugen, H., & Diederich, M. (2016e). Returning home. Retrieved from https://uturnasia.com/2016/01/22/returning-home/
Haugen, H., & Diederich, M. (2016f). Imagining a future. Retrieved from https://uturnasia.com/2016/01/20/aspirations/
Kipnis, A. (2007). Neoliberalism reified: Suzhi discourse and tropes of neoliberalism in the People's Republic of China. *Journal of the Royal Anthropological Institute*, *13*, 383–400.
Kleinman, A., Yan, Y., Jun, J., Lee, S., Zhang, E., Tianshu, P., Jinhau, G. (Eds.). (2011). *Deep China: The moral life of the person: What anthropology and psychiatry tell us about China today*. Berkeley, CA: University of California Press.
Kundera, M. (2005). *The unbearable lightness of being*. New York, NY: HarperCollins.
Morais, I. (2009). Chinese "Wahala": The tribulations of Nigerian "Bushfallers" in a Chinese territory. *Journal of Global Cultural Studies*, *5*, 2–22.
Munz, R., & Ulrich, R. (2004). Changing patterns of immigration to Germany, 1945–1997. Retrieved from https://migration.ucdavis.edu/rs/more.php?id=69
Oishi, N. (2012). The limits of immigration policies: The challenges of highly skilled migration in Japan. *American Behavioral Scientist*, *20*(10), 1–21.
Said, E. (1993). Intellectual exile: Expatriates and marginals. *Grand Street*, *47*, 112–124.
Selvon, S. (1989). *The lonely Londoners*. London, UK: Longmans.
Spencer, I. (1997). *British immigration policy since 1939*. Abingdon, UK: Routledge.
Strenger, C. (2013). The new cosmopolitans: Challenges and discontents. *Psychoanalytic Psychology*, *30*(2), 264–280.
Tsolidis, G. (2014). Introduction. In G. Tsolidis (Ed.), *International perspectives on migration, diaspora and identity: Cross-national experiences* (pp. 1–18). Dordrecht: Springer.

2 Self in the World

Self-construction in the twenty-first century is both a daunting and an exhilarating task. Individuals face complex forces, such as a rampant capitalism, its dominant market ethos, and its globalizing mechanisms that seek to homogenize and pacify them. Yet at the same time, potentially reflective and autonomous individuals have access to a diverse range of healthy ways of thinking about being in the world. This enables them to mobilize internal resources and access external resources that facilitate their ability to sculpt selves that are ethical, productive, and caring. A feature of the complexity of the settings in which people are embedded is its lack of fixity, a degree of liquidity that presents both opportunity and risk and generates much ambivalence (Bauman, 1991, 2001).

Psychological sophistication that develops, in part as a result of support from rich networks can in turn facilitate substantive self-development. Correspondingly, the act of self-construction can involve acknowledging and cultivating multiple self-states. This in turn engenders a sense of comfort with hybrid combinations of those self-states and the ability to also tolerate tension between them, as they can, at times, be in conflict with each other (Mitchell, 1993). Such conflict arises from the fluidity of opportunities, rising levels of anxiety, inequality, and increasing resistance to aspects of modernity.

In doing such work, individuals often yearn for some degree of ontological certainty, even as they take pleasure in discovering and developing heretofore unacknowledged or unknown aspects of the self. Given the myriad contingencies they must manage, including themselves as sources and subjects of contingency, there is an urgency and riskiness to this self-work in settings that range from the hostile but seductive, to the indifferent, and to the attractive. At the same time, I would argue that the opportunity to be challenged, albeit with some risk, is a motivating factor for individuals.

To complicate matters further, settings where self-construction and managing self-states occur are themselves in flux and contain the possibilities of both opportunity and risk. The modern economy increasingly offers opportunities for creative workers to excel, but at the same time, it increases the level of risk as the suite of skills in demand is forever changing. So, for example, whereas basic computer coders were once in high demand, that role is ever so slowly being commodified (Bureau of Labor Statistics, 2017a), with instead, an increase in demand for software developers, a job demanding a high level of creativity in addition to coding skills (Bureau of Labor Statistics, 2017b).

Economic factors and the anxieties and dreams they elicit, among other factors, influence self-construction and drive migration (Beltsiou, 2016). In part due to the challenges and attendant anxieties of constructing the self and the wish to be mobile, as exemplified by migration. So an enhanced sense of mobility is increasingly a factor in how a modern individual constructs their sense of self (Beltsiou, 2016). Such mobility speaks to relocating to a setting that would facilitate self-development work, given the difficulty in doing such work at home.

The increasingly transnational style of relating to family and friends, using multimedia platforms, makes the individual aware of an expanding array of ways of understanding the world and ways of being in the world. The idea of the self and the possibilities for agency become increasingly expansive and fluid. These are enhanced by the reflective capabilities of the individual attuned to both opportunity and risk.

In summary, such self-work is reflective of the uniquely human attempt to find meaning, be authentic, exercise agency, and be recognized as special in diverse and fluid contexts that can hopefully validate the sense of self. These issues are explored in part through the experiences of Africana workers in China.

Vignette: Elaine, an Africana Teacher in China

About Elaine

Elaine is a 32-year-old Afro-Jamaican woman who has been living in China for the past 8 years. She has a postgraduate degree in international communications from a European university with a Chinese campus, where the instruction was in English. She is a full-time lecturer in English at a Chinese university in a medium-sized city close to Shanghai.

Elaine grew up in a middle-class home in Jamaica with both parents; her mother is an educator, and her father works in property management. Her younger sister is a graduate student in the physical sciences. Elaine's parents encouraged their children to travel and took out loans to facilitate their studying and traveling abroad, a generous act that allowed Elaine to study and live in Panama for a year prior to going to university. Elaine noted, "My parents took out a loan so I could go. It was the best year of my life. I felt free in relation to my family."

While Elaine is very appreciative of the sacrifices her parents made that enabled her and her sister to expand their perceptions of the world, she is also attuned to the fact that their sacrifice allowed her to experience the joy of being away from them given their conservative and at times restrictive child-rearing ethos.

Professional Bleakness of Home and Restraints of Parents vs. Sense of Home as Familiar and Always Available

Elaine portrays her parents as being religiously conservative and as often selectively limiting her ability to explore and develop as an individual within the home and the tight-knit community in which she lived. Upon completion of her undergraduate degree, Elaine could not find work that paid well and was intellectually challenging. "It was mostly part-time work [in Jamaica]. I was able to get a visa to work in the United Kingdom. I like to travel, am curious about other cultures."

On her regular trips back home, she enjoys the familiarity and pleasures of friends, food, and places, but she still experiences home as limiting: "Money stretches farther in China. It would be difficult to explore the world using Jamaica as a base. … In Jamaica, there is a high cost of living. Within China there are diverse cultural experiences."

Elaine appears to be ambivalent about some aspects of her development, which results in her dreaming and yet holding herself back. So while she has attained an advanced degree in international relations, she has made no substantive attempts to pursue work opportunities in this area. Coming to China was supposed to have forced her to be more professionally adventurous, but she notes rather wryly that she has chosen to live in relatively conservative places and has not grasped challenging opportunities that have come her way. Elaine attributes her ambivalence in part to her conservative upbringing, in that it seems to constrain her from being bold and innovative.

Professional Attractions of China vs. Home-Related Limits on Elaine's Socio-Emotional Development

With assistance from family and peers abroad, Elaine spent 2 years working in the United Kingdom, where she also attained qualifications in teaching English as a second language. Given the paucity of professional opportunities at home, Elaine inquired of peers and family members in the Jamaican diaspora about working abroad. She concluded that the career prospects in the United States and Canada were much like those in England: opportunities that did not excite her and would not contribute to much personal growth.

One person mentioned a friend who had gone to China and was excited by the life she was living there:

> I wanted a very different cultural experience, so I did not do South America. There were opportunities in Asia, Korea, Japan, and

> China. Japan was my first choice as I had studied the language, but there were few openings. China was hosting the Olympics and had a big role in the world. ... I have always been curious and liked to travel, so when I heard there were job opportunities in China, I decided to check it out.

Elaine searched online, was offered a university-level job teaching English, and traveled to China alone. She was aware of the risks of the move, but she knew that she could return home at any time that she wished and so proceeded undaunted. She was the first Black person to live in the town where she was placed, residing with other non-Chinese faculty who also taught English.

Over time, Elaine moved to other small Chinese cities as a teacher, cities she usually selected for their relative proximity to Shanghai or Beijing, major transportation hubs, that allowed her to indulge in her passion for travel. Shanghai also has an organized Caribbean community mostly of highly skilled and credentialed Africana professionals working in the areas of teaching, finance, business, and design. It provides networking opportunities, access to Black hair stylists, and dating opportunities. Elaine, from a perspective of unblinking love for her home country, was clear that it offered none of the opportunities that she imagined pursuing abroad.

Professional Attractions of China vs. Personal Losses of Living in China

In her home city, Elaine socializes mostly with expatriate teachers and is generally wary in her relationships with Chinese nationals. She says:

> You have to be careful. They will get close to you to know what you are doing, but not because they are genuine. They will report you if you break a rule; cleaning person reports your activities and possessions to the landlord, and they are rewarded for reporting.

Such wariness concerning people she has met in China extends to romantic areas of her life. While she would like to marry, Elaine despairs of what she perceives as the transient and at times promiscuous lifestyles of the men in the Shanghai Africana community. She lacks any interest in Chinese men. "Chinese men are not assertive. They will not approach you directly. It is easier for foreign men to date Chinese women than the other way round," she says. Despite these concerns, she has developed genuine and mutually gratifying relationships with a few Chinese nationals, most of whom have lived and traveled abroad.

At the same time, she is not overly enamored regarding her relations with her expatriate peers: "I have to be careful who I socialize with, as some are inconsiderate and will exploit my tendency to be very helpful. So, in some ways, they are no different from some of the Chinese people I have to deal with."

Risks of Self-Making in China

Elaine was confronted with repeated acts of racism in China that were both discomforting and growth enhancing:

> I was qualified for a teaching position but was explicitly rejected because I was not White. They would give an English language teaching position to a non-native English speaker such as a Russian. There is a Ukrainian guy who gets so many more job offers than he could possibly accept, even though his English is not as good as mine. If you are Black and you have an American or a British passport, you will get more job offers than Black people from Africa and the Caribbean. If you are White, you will not lack for work.

Elaine is clear that there is a definite privileging of Whiteness in Chinese culture that drives these racist acts:

> White is next to God. There are a lot of skin products with whitening agents. They fix their eyes (surgically) to get the double fold. They look down on their eyes. I am much more race-conscious and aware of the fact that I am Black. I took a while to realize that I was not just a foreigner but was also Black. The small city that I was living in had not seen many foreigners. It took a while to get used to the staring, and then I realized that I stood out. I did not feel that way when I lived in Panama.

Alongside coping with racism, Elaine views Chinese preoccupation with materialism and unethical business practices as widespread:

> While I always have to be on my guard, I also have to be careful to maintain my own values. It is easy to get into rude behavior with the Chinese such as shouting and shoving. I have learned to pick my battles.

These risks fuel her ambivalence, which in turn makes her very careful to select work sites that will facilitate her living a reasonably enjoyable life.

Opportunities for Self-Making in China

Living in China has provided myriad opportunities for her to grow further as a person. Elaine enjoys the salary; she is able to save for her retirement, financially assist family members, and travel extensively. She perceives herself as a more thoughtful person, and she feels autonomous and more resilient. She has a greater sense of her ethnic identity, which has enabled her to develop a more tolerant and sophisticated worldview: "I got my masters, and I am much more open-minded. I am better able to see things from a non-Western perspective."

Ambivalence as a Feature of Self-Making in China

Living and working in China often generates mixed feeling states, and this ambivalence is often evident in Elaine's life, such as in the area of spirituality. Elaine intermittently attends religious services in her hometown, which exposes her to more positive aspects of Chinese culture in a community of like-minded people. She does note, however, that the state-mandated generic nature of the services often leaves her spiritually unfulfilled.

Ongoing Uncertainty Regarding Long-Term Goals and Available Opportunities

While Elaine is clear that she will not settle permanently in China, she has doubts as to whether she could ever find well-paying and meaningful work at home: "I can always go back, and I will probably retire there, but right now, I can't make a living there," Elaine says. She feels that she needs to commit to building a career, but as of yet is uncertain as to what it might be:

> Every year I say it is my last year, but the world-wide job situation is bad. It is not great in China, but I can take a trip annually. I am still job hunting and hope to stop teaching and do something more in line with my studies.

Elaine has not ruled out the possibility of working in Europe or North America. This idea of being peripatetic is a source of excitement and opportunity, as well as unsettling confusion, again reflecting an ambivalent stance in major areas of her life.

The Self and Identifications: Recognition

Recognition and positive validation are important interpersonal goals, and individuals will attempt to deploy aspects of the self that facilitate such recognition. While this speaks to a multiplicity of self-features, some constantly changing in the light of new contingencies, the individual perceives the self as being fairly constant. For such complex self-management—involving bringing an array of different aspects of the self to the forefront, while also maintaining an overall coherence of self for oneself—to be effective, a degree of insight and robust agency is necessary. Given the abundance of choices available, the swiftness of change, and the absence of any definitive guidelines, the individual needs to be thoughtful about how he or she exercises agency and what aspects of the self to present in a given situation.

Bodomo (2012) observed how many North Africans are careful not to refer to themselves as Africans in China, while a Canadian man of Caribbean heritage stated to me that he does not correct Chinese peers who assume that he is African American. In the first instance, within the category of Blackness in China, African is perceived as low status, while African American has high status. A poor ability to thoughtfully manage identity fluidity can lead to costly errors or missed opportunities.

A certain degree of identity fluidity, as well as the deployment of different aspects of one's identity, are prominent features of the modern self and are especially evident, in those like Elaine, engaging in transnational work.

Elaine engages in successful identity management, as demonstrated in her approach to maintaining cordial relationships with Chinese people, while not revealing too much of herself unless the person proves very trustworthy. She must be vigilant given that some forms of self-disclosure could benefit them but be costly to her. Elaine adopts a similar approach with many of her non-Chinese peers, given a similar predilection to exploit her.

The process of living abroad as an exercise in self-improvement changes how individuals perceive themselves and their home country. Such changes can be a source of ambivalence, as is evident within Elaine who is proud of her identifications with home and yet now realizes that she has no desire in the foreseeable future to live there again, given its constraints. So, there is both joy about home and melancholy, given its limited ability to support self-development.

Elaine has some appreciation of the need to be tolerant, to feel heightened vigilance with regard to being protective and efficient and joy in achievements, alongside a melancholic stance with regard to the elusiveness of home. It is, however, a challenge for her to hold vigilance, joy, and melancholia in productive tension. At times, she reports feeling "all over the map," uncertain as how to think and feel.

Migration

Trends

Migration, defined as crossing borders in flight from home or in search of work, is increasing, with an estimated 244 million migrants in 2015 (Menozzi, 2016). Some are immigrants; while others, such as Elaine, are seeking work with no interest to reside permanently in the host country. There is a worldwide demand for talented and highly credentialed workers, including those from the Africana world (Balogun,

2011). Many, such as health care workers, academics, computer technology experts, and engineers, are granted permanent residency in the developed countries.

In much of Asia, and increasingly in other parts of the world, there is a rise in the amount of long-term foreign workers who either do not intend to live permanently in the host country or will never be allowed to do so. This growing population includes workers from the Indian and African continents working in the Gulf States and Saudi Arabia, along with Filipinos in Hong Kong and Africana persons in China.

One subgroup of these foreign workers has been dubbed the *new cosmopolitans* (Strenger, 2013). Eternally peripatetic in response to a demand for their scarce and lucratively remunerated services, and speaking English, home for many of them appears to be wherever they are. Elaine is clearly embedded in such a group, with a mostly Western-oriented social group of friends and colleagues. Within the Africana community in China, this group includes teachers in the global network of international primary and secondary schools and faculty in tertiary institutions. It also includes administrators at the executive level, human resources specialists, information technology workers, and persons skilled at sales and marketing.

They go where the work is and do not perceive themselves as full-fledged members of the host culture, due in part to its hostile immigration policies. This also speaks in part to their attachment to the lifestyle of a sojourner, who, while anchored psychologically, if somewhat ambivalently, to a sense of belonging linked to some aspect of the home culture, does not need to actually live there. Many maintain strong, if at times ambivalent, relationships to their home country as is evident in the case of Elaine.

Then there are the undocumented and often low-skilled workers, some of whom die trying to achieve their aspirations, while others simply move from one site of immobility to another (Haugen, 2012; Haugen & Diederich, 2016a, 2016b, 2016c, 2016d, 2016e, 2016f). By definition, their numbers are unknown, as are their outcomes, given the necessity of avoiding official scrutiny. They comprise all known national, ethnic, racial, gender, and religious groupings. Some, given the prominence of their social markers, such as pigmentation, gender, and language, are more noticeable than others. As a result, these workers are more vulnerable to exploitation and incarceration.

Psychodynamics of the Skilled and Ambivalent: A New Subgroup of Foreign Workers

Elaine exemplifies the psychodynamics of a significant subgroup of twenty-first-century migrants, who can be thought of as skilled and ambivalent. She, like so many of her peers and others, must leverage her skill sets to migrate, however temporarily, to a place that will adequately remunerate her for her skills and allow her to explore and engage in fruitful and not too costly self-development.

The move to China, through the market recognition of Elaine's skills, enhances her self-worth, increases her capabilities, broadens her worldview, expands her sense of agency, and increases her material wealth. She is however, socially isolated, and she struggles to make sense of her long-standing ambivalences around being assertive and her concerns regarding intimacy and spirituality. Elaine's lack of Chinese language fluency compounds her difficulties in establishing a diverse set of mutually nurturing relationships where she can work on these issues. As a result, China, like her home country, is experienced with a degree of ambivalence.

Another Reason for Ambivalence: Market Forces in the Personal Realm

Elaine exemplifies an approach to self-construction that reflects both curiosity and caution around substantive chance-taking. In China, such an approach is consistent with a market ethos and political ideology that encourages materiality and technical intellect but is wary of substantive approaches to self-development that focus on rights demand, spirituality, and community. The emphasis on consumption fuels the market demand for increased production of goods and services. It also satisfies the political goal of attempting to shift the individual's focus away from political concerns about issues of governance and accountability.

While she is financially comfortable, Elaine is not preoccupied with the material. She has not invested substantially in the social aspect given her long-standing ambivalence around intimacy and her experiences in China. This is evident in her residing at some distance from a diverse English-speaking community and is indicative of her wariness around relating substantially, a position that she acknowledges predated her coming to China. Elaine was socialized to focus on cognitive achievements with a view to career development and a concomitant marginalization of the thoughtful cultivation of the intimate and the social. This is reflective of the neoliberal ethos in her home country, where personal development is yoked to the demands of the marketplace. In such a setting, one is always being ranked and quantified, and this might well have influenced Elaine's attitude to Chinese persons.

One pleasure derived but probably not consciously acknowledged by Elaine is that she is materially much better off than the average Chinese person. This might be especially gratifying given that this would not have been the case in Jamaica in relation to the more affluent Chinese Jamaican community there. So in either country using a market metric she is not on equal footing with the person of Chinese heritage, ending up relatively alone and deriving some austere pleasure alongside a sense of something lacking from that position.

Powerful market forces have influenced both how Elaine has been socialized and her self-fashioning work. This results in her appearing to be in a perpetual transitional space, attempting to assuage a sense of what has been called "in-between-ness" (Conway, 2007), experiencing strong feelings of not quite belonging at home or in China. She perceives both sites as sources of substantive frustration and of similar limits, and she doesn't feel quite at home in either place, yet she derives complementary gratifications from both. The resulting dynamic has a feeling of shopping for the components of a self and not quite finding all of them. The challenge then for Elaine, and others in this state of in-between-ness, is to find ways of adaptively managing the ambivalence it yields, this sense of always not quite belonging. They must juggle the gratifications alongside the unease that this state engenders in them.

The Market and the Self

Aspects of the Self Valued by the Market

Self-worth is sustained in part by a sense of competence that is derived from cognitively oriented work and emotionally oriented relating. Increasingly in neoliberal cultures, self-worth is primarily defined in terms of being successful in relation to a capitalist market manifested as the presentation to the market of passions, vulnerabilities, potentials, and capabilities (Kipnis, 2007). The market emphasis on commodification, quantification, consumption, and production narrows the definition of the self (Strenger, 2016). Strenger also argues that we are inherently vulnerable to find such a system attractive given our fear of being unacknowledged and having to deal with uncertainty. McGowan (2016) complements this point by noting the relentless pursuit and elusiveness of satisfaction in capitalist-oriented market cultures. Reducing all aspects of self-worth to being acquisitive and to quantitative and seemingly objective metrics unwittingly narrows down the range of features of self-worth that is deemed important.

Interests that make us richly human such as "being-for-the other" (Levinas, 1985, p. 96) define the self as always in a relationship of healthy interdependence. This would be manifested as participation in religious and community activities, commitments that are often marginalized by market values. Among low-income Africana traders in Guangzhou attending non-state-sanctioned churches, Haugen (2012) noted a market-inflected sermonizing that coaches worshipers in how to achieve and manage material success, often promising that some supernatural entity will facilitate them acquiring wealth. Here, religious activities are utilitarian, sculpted to be in the service of wealth creation.

This profit-oriented ethos influences all participants in the market, resulting in potential objectification of individuals by rewarding only those aspects of their productive self that can consume and can generate a surplus. So, in Elaine's case, the Chinese market for English teachers places a high premium on English language competency when combined with the presence of Caucasian physical phenotypes among those offering those services. As a result Elaine (who is Black) earns less relative to a teacher with Caucasian features.

In the absence of desired skill sets, some Africana workers in China live precarious lives, exacerbated by them being embedded in networks that lack the information set and material and political resources necessary to effectively compete and generate attractive surpluses (Haugen, 2012; Haugen & Diederich, 2016a, 2016b, 2016c, 2016d, 2016e, 2016f). In addition to being financially impoverished, some who have tied their self-worth to market standards experience themselves as unsuccessful.

This over-privileging of cognitive skill sets can lead to a peripatetic lifestyle as individuals seek ever-higher return on their intellectual capital (Strenger, 2016). Such an approach can contribute to weak attachment ties to others and to community, resulting in a dissociated aspect of self that can engender feelings of depression and alienation. Such individuals, many in search of the next big opportunity, eschew long-term commitments and emotional attachments. This is evident with Elaine, who has scores of attachments to individuals across the globe but paradoxically considers very few of them to be substantial friends.

Marginalized Aspects of the Self

Such a stance that constructs self-worth as tightly linked to market values can also work against the creation of diverse and supportive communities, an issue that Elaine and many others find challenging. Given the high-value attached to intellectual achievement, this often makes them not quite fit in wherever they reside. They are invariably critical of the place and are therefore less accepted by the members of the communities in which they are embedded (Strenger, 2013). They are often oblivious to the paradox inherent in the fact that the lack in the local, which they bemoan, generates the demand that they are generously remunerated for fulfilling. This incuriosity, if not disdain, makes them oblivious to the local's strengths that are not market mediated.

Therefore, alongside a sense of themselves as being overachievers is an often-accompanying loneliness that persists: "Because they do not feel that they safely belong to their groups, they will tend to feel exposed and vulnerable for the rest of their lives. They are never sure that the dominant group will not turn against them" (Strenger, 2013, p. 272). They have more opportunities but are accompanied by more anxieties and are therefore vulnerable not just to the gyrations of the global economy, but also to the vicissitudes of local sentiment. As a consequence, there is always an irreducible sense of *otherness*, anxiety, and loneliness. Africana workers who are not fluent in Chinese have a limited and transient pool of potential friends, making it challenging to develop ongoing relationships. They must also cope with the anxiety generated by the seemingly arbitrary and ever-changing rules of annual visa renewal requirements.

Market-Generated Ambivalence

Capitalism is a multifaceted system of surplus generation and accumulation and accomplishes this in part by masking where the individual's true desire lies.

> The capitalist regime produces subjects who cling feverishly to the image of their own dissatisfaction and thus to the promise, constantly made explicit in a capitalist society, of a way to escape the dissatisfaction through either accumulation of capital or the acquisition of commodity.
>
> (McGowan, 2016, p. 11)

What matters is the promise, and hidden from the consumer, the failure, to achieve its ultimate complete satisfaction. This of course is predicated on a sense of dissatisfaction with the present state of affairs, a sense of lack that the investment of time and resources will assuage.

It is a system that is conflictual, exploitive, and anxiety producing, alongside being a system that offers opportunities for creativity, enhanced agency, and the achievement of well-being. It can therefore be thought of as a major source of ambivalence that all modern individuals struggle to adaptively manage (Hermans & Dimaggio, 2007). Conflict often arises as the individual seeks to curtail the soul-destroying aspects of capitalism calibrated an overly exploitive market ethos. At the same time, Nandy (1998b) notes that capitalism through the globalization process disseminates a way for the creation and sustainability of a holistic self. Such potential liberatory perspectives question the tempting myth of the individual as unfettered and having reasonable and equal access to the resources necessary to love and work in meaningful ways. There is a growing awareness that the system is rigged and that, although it might well offer opportunities, there are also considerable and often insurmountable obstacles to access, and for some the increasing possibility of been limited to harvesting immobility and bitterness.

For some people, capitalism can act as an incentive to take up thoughtful initiatives that they hold in tension with the awareness of constraints, thereby fueling ambivalence as an inoculation against either an overly heady optimism or a crippling despair. Here, capitalism in its ever protean fashion creates a space, albeit a highly conditional one, in China that addresses the need to belong and to exercise agency in the service of assuaging desire. China's insatiable demand for talented individuals with creative skills resulted in it creating a special visa class for such individuals and on occasion granting them permanent residency. Stephon Marbury is an African American celebrated basketball star in the Chinese leagues who was granted permanent residency, one of only 5,000 granted to over 600,000 foreigners residing in China (Zhao, 2015). One way of understanding this is for individuals to acknowledge that the self must always be sensitive to the transactional demands and costs of living in a world of globalized capitalism and that they must build the capabilities necessary to both develop and protect the self, while adaptively managing the inherent ambivalence that such work generates. This ambivalence is fueled by the paradox that manifests itself in pursuing the satisfaction of desire even while accepting the inevitable limits on the degree to which it will be assuaged (McGowan, 2016).

Ambivalence is a long-standing concept in psychoanalysis (Freud, 1961), and stipulates that feeling, thought, or act triggers both desire and gratification, alongside frustration and possible withdrawal. Ambivalence thrives in late modernity given the uncertainty of how to act and the costliness and inevitable sense of dissatisfaction in seeking to assuage desire. Individuals pursue satisfaction despite its ultimate elusiveness and the healthy necessity to come to terms with accepting some degree of dissatisfaction as inevitable.

By way of example, the Africana person is ambivalent about home: It is a site of many treasured gratifications, especially in the interpersonal and aesthetic realms, yet it is also a site of many frustrations experienced in the pursuit of attempts to develop professionally and to acquire wealth. A mirror image of ambivalence occurs in China, where some gratification is derived in the cognitive and material realms, while needs for recognition, belonging, and community are often frustrated. In both situations, what is desired and what is unattractive are coupled, and the individual must develop adaptive ways to manage the ensuing ambivalence.

Given that fluidity and uncertainty are prominent features of a capitalist-driven neoliberalism, ambivalence abounds and calls for healthy adaptations by the individual. As Botticelli (2004) notes, sensitivity as to how misery is introjected into the psyche through the social unconscious might, if insightfully managed, allow individuals to separate out their own conflicts and the misery they yield from those conflicts that are imported. Recognizing the impossibility of being completely satisfied is a critical feature of adaptive ambivalence. It allows for healthy defenses that could contain such introjects, while mobilizing to grasp opportunity, while always holding both in tension.

Self

Possibilities and Risks

The combination of the emergence of a multiplicity of ways of being in the world and the potentially increased agency derived from that allows the individual some latitude in self-construction acts (Bauman, 2001). These advantages, ushered in by the ethos of modernity, offer the possibility to pursue and present ways of being that are authentic and fulfilling in the individual's attempts to love and work in the world. At the same time, the decline in authoritative and constraining epistemologies alongside the dominance of a market ethos, places the individual at risk for living an often false, shallow, and ultimately ungratifying life. Individuals therefore find themselves in a place of uncertainty that offers both risk and reward, but with no definitive way of limiting the first or of increasing the possibility of the second. The challenge is then to fashion a self that can manage the vicissitudes of modernity by embracing limits on the degree of satisfaction that can be attained (McGowan, 2016). This is a healthy defense against the sense of despair that results from the futile pursuit of a sense of being completely satisfied.

The modern individual increasingly must manage the tensions between the idea of the self as integrated and consistent and the notion of a self that is fractious, multifaceted, and ever-changing in response to relational demands and needs (Mitchell, 1993). In his disquisition on the self, Mitchell (1993) embeds its development in a challenging cultural environment:

> What does it mean to be a person? What sort of persons are we? How are we connected and related to each other? This sort of self-reflection has become a preoccupying concern: on a global level, in the face of self-contamination and self-annihilation; on an international level, in the wake of astounding shifts in the way nations are positioning themselves vis-à-vis each other; on a national level, in the context of shrinking economic and political horizons; and on an individual level in the wake of historically unprecedented shifts in social, economic, and gender roles.
>
> (p. 100)

Such changes might well grant individuals more leeway with regard to self-constructing, albeit with more anxiety given the stress of complexity and uncertainty.

Ways of Thinking About the Self: Multiplicity of Self-States

There are two seemingly opposed, psychoanalytically informed ideas as to how to think about the meaning of self. One speaks to the self as single, private, stable, consistent across time, integrated, existing in layers that are not all readily, consciously accessible. The second model speaks to the self as multiple, relational, discontinuous, and inherently conflictual (Mitchell, 1993). Grinberg and Grinberg (1982) subscribe to the first perspective, as they portray the self as continuity and sameness and therefore as relatively unchanging.

Mitchell (1993) has written in depth on both of these perspectives and makes the following core points. With regard to the self as singular and continuous, he links this to the idea of a spatial metaphor as articulated in Freud's structural model. This approach portrays the mind and the resultant psychic operations as a multi-layered space, not unlike an onion with the self at its core. This self has some degree of autonomy given that individuals exercise some control regarding who has access to their thoughts and affects. This approach, with its sense of separateness and obscuring, does not stress the relational requirements of the self.

The Relational Self

The paradox in this view of the self as autonomous and private, however, is that the self is intrinsically relationally inclined. The more we delve into the private self, the more we are connected to others who have facilitated us becoming a self. "We rely on both self-reflection and the reflection from others to define ourselves with the former speaking to a unique and private perspective," Mitchell (1993, p. 113) says.

In reality, the self is discontinuous; it is a multiplicity of self-states and is best understood through a temporal metaphor. According to Mitchell (1993),

> Selves are what people do and experience over time rather than something that exists somewhere. Self refers to the subjective organization of meanings one creates as one moves through time doing things, such as having ideas and feelings, including some self-reflective feelings about oneself.
>
> (pp. 101–102)

While the individual, for adaptive reasons, maintains the essential fiction of the self as continuous and relatively unchanging, a dispassionate view reveals a self that has a multiplicity of ways of presenting a diverse range of self-states, all of which are never consciously present, and a self that changes and transforms over time.

Partly as a function of the demands of relating, some self-states are prominent, while others are more subordinate. So, for some Africana persons in China, much thought goes into finding safe ways of asserting the political self, the aspects that speak to advocacy. The Africana merchants in Yiwu working with a receptive municipal administration have jointly developed effective mechanisms to resolve business related concerns (Cisse, 2015). These merchants must keep a tight rein on those aspects of the self that would seek expression through advocating for more substantive systemic changes, a stance that would not be entertained by the Chinese authorities.

As a consequence, a given relationship can be examined from different self-perspectives, with each self-state having its own history of interacting within that particular relationship, thus contributing to some discontinuity. "Because we learn to become a person through interactions with different others and through different kinds of interactions with the same other, our experience of self is discontinuous, composed of different configurations, different selves with different others" (Mitchell, 1993, p. 104). Some Africana traders report being quite wary of business relationships based solely on ethnic similarity due to having been exploited by their own; they focus, instead, on trustworthiness regardless of ethnic affinity.

Dynamic Self-States

Another approach that may be useful in thinking about the self would speak to self-states as dynamic, not all being rational, and with some being dissociative. Other self-states are mostly unconscious, often conflictual, always negotiating, with all optimally constituting a turbulent if whole self (Bromberg, 1996). Given such a dynamic intrapsychic process in the context of tumultuous cultural settings, the self can be said to always carry some degree of ambivalence toward both its ways of being and toward the various socio-emotional relationships in which it is embedded. Some Africana women in China report pleasure at being part of a diverse Africana community, but at the same time, they are wary of Africana men, saying that many of them are quite patriarchal in their approach to gendered relationships. The push to relate sits alongside a healthy wariness given the history of dissatisfaction and hurt.

A relational push is motivated by a strong desire for recognition and its attendant benefits. Strenger (2016) argues that recognition, alongside the fear of its opposite, insignificance, animates how the individual engages the world. Such recognition bolsters self-esteem and is gained by being embedded in networks that offer the appropriate tutoring and others that recognize, utilize, and reward the capabilities being offered. A significant portion of migration broadly defined is motivated by a quest for self-development, the acquisition of capabilities, and a broadened worldview resulting in a quality of recognition and agency not possible at home. Their appropriate management of the quest for healthy recognition allows individuals to be more dynamic and fluid in how they deploy self-states in contrast to the constraints experienced at home.

Self and Otherness

Also integral to any sense of the modern self is managing an irreducible sense of *otherness* and the ambivalence that comes from not quite fitting in. This can develop as a result of choice or of an externally imposed fiat resulting in an individual attempting to find adaptive ways to manage these states. Such self-work is facilitated by being embedded in multiple networks, in each of which there is both inevitably gratification and validation, alongside varying degrees of a lack of fit and the attendant sense of being limited. So there is always some degree of a sense of disconnectedness, aloneness, and otherness.

Given these self-features, the argument has been made that a stable substantively gratified, and singular sense of self is an illusion in the modern world, in which the assumption of mastery and the attainment of certainty and complete satisfaction is impossible (Bauman, 2001; McGowan, 2016; Mitchell, 1993). The challenge is to seek new ways of understanding and healthily managing the expression of desire and the need for recognition. Individuals therefore pursue meaning, even while accepting the elusiveness of complete understanding.

Given the less than seamless integrating of the various self-states, there is space to make tentative alliances and ambivalent liaisons in the service of achieving some desired goal. This resonates with Bromberg's (1996) assertion that "health is the ability to stand in the spaces between realities without losing any of them; the capacity to feel like one self while being many" (p. 512). Here lies the possibility of creating a subjective sense of stability and meaning-making alongside an awareness of its contingent nature.

Development, Culture, and Self

Diversity of the Self and of Culture

The self in all its diversity is always embedded in a multiplicity of cultural settings that influence the self and over time are influenced by the self. Until quite recently, most psychoanalytic theories have not focused on the sociopolitical perspectives on self-development, on how the social unconscious is an influential factor in how various self-states develop, and on the conditions that facilitate or inhibit their expression of said self-states. The social unconscious reflects the sum total of cultural factors that influence ways of thinking, feeling, and acting outside of the individual's conscious awareness (Hopper, 2002). So, for example, often many Africana persons are exposed to a migration narrative supportive of going abroad to further self-development. Such a narrative is comprised of the stories of family members, multimedia images of "abroad," and the material benefits accruing to the families in the home country sent by those who have migrated. These factors might not be consciously acknowledged or weaved together, but nevertheless, they might well bias the person to think of leaving home as a good idea.

Traditional relational models tend to focus on interpersonal relationships while marginalizing the impact of larger social forces on how self-states develop and how they might be privileged or marginalized. To the degree that such forces are acknowledged as an intrapsychic imperative, it is with the expectation that individuals curb impulses that threaten the ordered and benign cultural setting in which they are embedded. Walls (2003) makes the point that the interpersonal is always cultural, and the various self-states are always influenced by and influencing social constructions such as gender, class, race, ethnicity, and religion among other factors in their diverse ways of presenting.

One must therefore take into consideration that contemporary cultures are quite diverse and therefore have spaces that facilitate the creation of equally diverse aspects of the self that cannot be reduced to the cultural profile of any one group. Given this possibility of multiple aspects of the self, hybrid self-states would be a consequence of subjective diversity and the particular intrapsychic operations that manage such diversity. The attempt to express any aspect of its various permutations would also be subject to the facilitating and constraining tendencies of the cultural contexts in which the individual is embedded. This, if well managed, contributes to a richer, more nuanced, albeit always ambivalent sense of self. The self in all its diversity is always embedded in a multiplicity of cultural settings that unconsciously influence thoughts and actions. At the same time, while influential, culture is also influenced by the self, a reality that is often overlooked.

The Social Unconscious and the Self

The term *social unconscious* is often associated with the writings of Earl Hopper (2002). Hopper argues that we are born into cultural settings that through political, educational, economic, religious, and other processes influence how we perceive the world; further, he states that these cultural settings facilitate and also restrain our agency. These perspectives, of which we are often unaware, constitute the social unconscious and profoundly influence how we define ourselves and how we relate to others. We are therefore not completely conscious masters of our psychic lives, given that we have internalized the perspectives of the cultural settings and relationships that sustain us. These perspectives generate both positive and negative emotions, but the individual may not necessarily make the link between these deep-seated influential factors and his or her more conscious experiences and actions.

So, some Africana persons come to China with long-standing and unexamined stereotypes about the Chinese derived from how they were socialized in their home countries. While they are outside of conscious awareness, such stereotypes do influence how Africana individuals feel, think, and act in their relationships with Chinese persons. This same pattern can be observed in relation to how some Chinese persons, think, feel, and act toward Africana individuals. The individual is not, however, a slave to these unconscious forces, as he also brings his own perspectives based on his predispositions, direct conscious experience, and reflective capacities. Some Africana traders challenge the deep-seated social belief that in a multicultural setting such as Guangzhou, their first obligation is to their ethnic kin. That is generally the default position, but some, on reflecting about their actual experiences, question such automatic obligation and instead are more consciously discerning and aware of the ways in which some of their kin have acted unethically toward them.

The social unconscious content can constrain individuals in ways that are healthy. Some Africana persons report that being in China has reinforced the importance of adhering to ethical principles learned long ago and often not consciously thought about. Confronted with unethical acts by some Chinese individuals, they are often tempted to respond in kind but find themselves uncomfortable contemplating acting in that way. These ways of thinking outside of consciousness can also constrain the individual from acting in ways that will enhance self-development. So some Africana persons are from cultures that have historically denigrated their ethnic Chinese populations, including their linguistic styles. This has made it difficult for some Africana persons to learn Chinese in China and therefore broaden their range of relationships.

Social Constraints on the Self

The influence of social forces can be very much in the service of oppression, of unethically constraining the individual (Fanon, 1967; Freire, 2000; Frosh, 2013). Elliot (2002) argues that aspects of the social unconscious align with the status quo and its unethical constraints on agency. This would be in contrast to internalizations that embrace the possibility of difference and the commonalities with other. Frosh (2013) notes a bias in mainstream psychodynamics of human dysfunction, where the fault lies within the individual who is unable to adhere to seemingly benign social norms. This point is emphasized and elaborated on by Fanon (1967), who was one of the first to explore the effects of the marginalization of colonized peoples' subjective world on the constitutionality of their psychic life. Gordon (2000), notes that Fanon argues that colonial subjectivities are exploited on the basis of both class and race. Schemes of rational explanation are here finding their limits. "In each instance, the black attempts to address a problem and encounters himself as a problem" (p. 33). Fanon (1967) further observes that for the subordinate individual, what is internalized as a guiding imperative in the social unconscious is often in the service of oppressing the individual rather than facilitating self-control. Such strictures hobble assertiveness and instead enforce obedience to mandates that limit self-development. In this formulation, oppressed individuals are socialized to believe that they are the source of their oppression, especially if they are of Africana heritage. Here, the expectation is one of obedience and passivity rather than reflection and assertiveness as an expression of their humanity. To analyze such individuals' pain from a purely psychological perspective is in fact to add to the oppression they are already experiencing due to a failure to acknowledge the influence of the interaction effects of capitalistic, gendered, and racist systems of dehumanization.

Many Africana persons are from former colonies or devalued minority communities where neocolonial attitudes persist and can be seen as the continuation of a history of a dedicated assault on assertiveness, pleasure, and spontaneity. The legacy of colonialism and neoliberalism is one of the individual being overly constrained so the oppressor's attempted monopoly over the realms of being human and agentic is very costly to challenge (Williams, 2016). For many such thwarted individuals, it is difficult to establish a psychological space of resistance and self-assertion.

While for many who are leaving home it is necessary to maintain psychological health and growth, the wish to be free coexists with internalized constraints on freedom. Nandy (1998b) observes that modern oppression is fought on the terrain of the intrapsychic, that it is "a battle between the dehumanized self and the objectified enemy, the technological bureaucrat and his reified victim, pseudo-rulers and their fearsome other selves projected unto their subjects" (p. 5). Through its near monopoly of media and curricula, the epistemology of oppression is continuously transmitted.

Therefore, one ought not to underestimate the substantive penetration of the mind by neocolonial and neoliberal epistemologies. In neocolonial contexts, there is a danger of internalizing the oppressor's marginalization and denigration of original attachments and worldviews, One is never outside of the oppressive epistemology, nor is one reduced to being one with it, hence Echeruo's (1999) observation of the lifelong influence of these epistemologies. This can result in a marginalizing of Africana perspectives and a resistance to this by Africana persons as they pursue their respective life projects.

Such projections are reflective of a negating stance toward the non-Western other, the marginalization of individual subjectivities, human rights, and attempts at self-development, Nandy (1998b) notes that, through its enlightenment project with its positivist techniques, the West appeared to demystify and marginalize non-Western frames of reference. Here, the goal was to establish hegemony of its own way of thinking and therefore devalue alternate epistemologies. What was constructed and contingent was adroitly presented as natural, normative, and unchanging.

Demystification can be thought of as emphasizing rational approaches to understanding all social phenomena and being skeptical of mystery, enchantment, and other subjective states that while giving meaning to the individual's life are not necessarily logical. The tendency from a positivist perspective is to deprecate and marginalize such modes of thought. For some Africana persons, being enchanted with some aspects of home serve as a buffer to aspects of the grounded and gritty reality of life in China. This is especially evident with regard to the spiritual and the emotional aspects of the individual (Nandy, 1998b). For the Africana person in China, there is a substantive risk that self-development can be limited to the development of the market-oriented intellectual capabilities that facilitate production, consumption, and an unwittingly also an emotional and spiritual lightness of being.

With differing and at times seemingly incompatible perspectives, the social unconscious is a site of conflict that generates some of the ambivalence that the individual experiences, and it also offers the potential of generating adaptive ways of responding. So as a consequence of its interactions with other components of the psyche, it becomes the site of not only conflict, but also of potentially adaptive compromise.

Multiplicity of Identifications: Ambivalences and Hybridities

An increasingly globalized world with its abundance of data offers individuals new ways of thinking about who they are and how to manage their multiplicity of identifications. These ways of being are accompanied by varying degrees of emotional attachment, and some aspects may well be in conflict within the self and between self and others. Globalization contributes to "partial identities" and "fragmented alliances" with their attendant anxieties (Copelman, in Akhtar, 1995, p. 1076), and it often creates conditions that result in individuals abandoning some identifications and adoption of others, resulting in their identity constellations often changing (Chun, 2009). For many Africana persons in China, there is a validation of some aspects of being with new identifications across ethnic and national boundaries and hybrid constructions functioning to encompass their cultural in-between-ness. These are all quite fluid and are selectively deployed, given the demands of a particular context and the resulting psychological turbulence can generate feelings of ambivalence.

At a minimum, within the long-standing identifications with the home cultures, there was some awareness that aspects of the self that had been thwarted and thus had fueled the decision to leave. In addition, there are equivalent tensions within the identifications with the host culture, given its less-than-unconditionally positive response to the foreigner. Individuals are therefore challenged to generate and sustain hybrid aspects of the self to meet the challenges of being in the host country.

Hybrid Identifications

These within and between cultural tensions often give rise to hybrid identity constructions that do not necessarily privilege unconditional identification with one group or place (Naujoks, 2010). One Afro-Caribbean man in China observed that his home was wherever he was and that while he was proud to be Black, he felt no need to identify with any given cultural space or group. Here, the definition of the self is less tied to necessarily being in a particular physical and social space.

Such hybridity around cultural identifications could have been in part made possible by growing up in diverse cultural settings in which there is a greater acceptance of poly vocality and especially of one's Africana heritage. In settings such as the large cosmopolitan cities of the United States and Europe, and the multi-ethnic African and Caribbean home cultures, there is a bias toward transculturalism and regionalism, alongside the accompanying ambiguities, contradictions, and ambivalences. Being socialized in such a setting creates the material for identity building that allows for openness to diverse ways of being and skepticism toward too strong an emphasis on a homogenizing sameness (Headley, 2011). Some Africana persons spoke of the pleasure in finding commonalities within difference such as being in a diverse community of folks who all identified as Africana and at the same time discovering cultural differences within that commonality.

One must therefore be wary of assuming undue fixity to cultural identifications or assuming that some essential identification is a given. One Africana foreign worker I spoke to in China is of Caribbean heritage, is a Canadian citizen, is a permanent resident of the United States, and is exploring the possibility of a long-term commitment to living in China. He thinks of himself as a Caribbean person but does not correct people who perceive him as an African American, as that classification has higher status in China than being a non-American Black.

Fluidity of Identities

Identity is therefore constituted not only by similarities, but also by differences regarding who we are and what we have become. This way of thinking about identity is one that points to the dynamics of change and an ongoing process of becoming that speaks to both the legacy of history and the possibilities of transformation within a given context of power (Hall, 2002). Given such potential fluidity, Hall stresses the importance of avoiding premature closure and also avoiding the impossible search for a final position that Scott (2005) refers to as "paradigm closure" (p. 8). This point is echoed by Grinberg and Grinberg (1982) when they speak of the need to be wary of attempting "a premature search for integration" (p. 8). They go on to note that

> At the same time that I confronted the problem of maintaining my identity, I struggled to change it, because when I de-idealized my task I could accept the "bad" aspects of my old culture and incorporate the "good" aspects of the new without completely renouncing my previous identifications.
>
> (p. 164)

Scott (2005) notes that such openness serves the purpose, "to draw us away from our consoling attachments to the idea of identity as imagined and lived as a continuous and developmentally unfolding of the self" (p. 13). While migrants and Africana workers in China may claim a core cultural identity, it is not necessarily faithful to an essentialized definition of that identity. Many hold in unconscious tension a tight embrace of that identity alongside variants, with some speaking to disenchantment and distancing.

Hierarchy and Deployment of Identifications

Immigrants and others away from home are therefore quite adept at building a self with a potentially shifting hierarchy of identifications and in bringing pragmatic and emotional considerations to bear as to which identifications are deployed at any given point in time, in the service of achieving mobility and agency (Bodomo, 2012). Such cultural code-switching is familiar to Africana individuals from culturally diverse settings. Bodomo (2012) noted this among some workers from North Africa who were careful never to identify themselves as Africans given the perceived negativity associated with that particular identity. It is also a necessary skill where a given presentation of some aspect of the self may not be prudent given its negative ascription by a dominant group. At other times it might be advantageous to assert a particular skill set. An example of this would be the interests in the intellectual aspects of the Africana individual by Chinese employers.

Such tactical deployment of identity, where possible, enhances the successful pursuit of agency, with the foreigner being thoughtful about which identities are privileged and which are marginalized. Given the demand for skilled and creative workers in China, some Africana workers will emphasize those aspects of their identity, given the sense of affirmation, agency, and mobility that it affords them. The richness and availability of identities is also a function in part of the cultural settings in which the individual is embedded. Already self-identifying at regional and national levels, some Afro-Caribbean workers in China report becoming increasingly aware of their African heritage (Adams, 2015). Consistent with Naujoks' (2010) typology, elements of personal, ethnic, regional, and diaspora factors contribute to the identity commitments of a given immigrant, and there is a unique calculus as to what aspects are deployed in a given context. Identity is therefore formed in the crucible of a multiplicity of struggles, psychological, social, and political in nature. This is what Scott (2005) refers to as a "war of position" (p. 6).

Identification and the Influence of the Political

The cultural networks in which the individual is embedded are by definition political, given their legitimate, and in some instances illegitimate, authority to facilitate and constrain various aspects of self-development and to accommodate the resulting agency. Speaking of Fanon's work, Fuss (1994) notes:

> Fanon's work also draws our attention to the historical and social conditions of identification. It reminds us that identification is never outside or prior to politics, that identification is always inscribed within a certain history: identification names not only the history of the subject but the subject in history. What Fanon gives us, in the end, is a politics that does not oppose the psychical but fundamentally presupposes it.
>
> (p. 39)

This is evident in the somewhat fluid ways in which some Chinese persons construct Africana identity. Many start from a place of a negative essentialized perspective. This can shift to a more positive construction often motivated by commercial interests.

So, the commercial center in Yiwu has ambitions of becoming a world-class trading center and creates the political space within which Africana businesspersons can bring more of themselves in terms of advocacy. This is in contrast to Guangzhou, where the authorities are less inclined to entertain identity claims around fairness and community obligations to their Africana businesspersons.

These spaces in which identity work is done are highly contested, and Stuart Hall (1990) speaks to this issue when he notes that:

> Cultural identities are the points of identification, the unstable points of identification or suture, which are made within the discourses of history and culture. Not an essence but a positioning. Hence, there is always a politics of identity, a politics of position, which has no absolute guarantee in an unproblematic, transcendental law of origin.
>
> (p. 226)

At the same time, one consequence of such political struggles is the creation of spaces for hybrid identities and/or re-feudalist moves in the service of belonging, given emotional needs and social context. No "pure" or uncontaminated ethnic identity exists in a globalized world. Given the antipathy toward peoples of Africana heritage among some Chinese people, Africana workers must reflect on how to effectively deploy competencies that will resonate with the needs of the Chinese marketplace, despite some negative ascriptions regarding their race or ethnicity. Such psychosocial frameworks therefore constitute limits to the idea of "sovereign agency" (Scott, 2005, p. 7). Individuals are therefore subject to "branded contingencies" (p. 7) that are both embodied, a feature of the physical aspects of culture, and are also social in nature. They constrain our capacity to act as culturally unencumbered and dispassionate creatures of pure reason exercising unconstrained agency (Scott, 2005).

The Challenges and Possibilities for Africana Self-Making

Challenges

Self-making in a time of uncertainty dominated by market-influenced identities is a project that requires resistance and re-significations. As Nandy (1998b) noted, there are opportunities with regard to possible and retrievable selves, providing one can manage the concomitant anxiety generated by the absence of definitive answers to ways of resolving conflict (Hermans & Dimaggio, 2007). The challenge of refashioning the self, elicits both excitement and anxiety.

Central to modern self-making are the challenges of recognition, of being affirmed as special, without necessarily paying too high a psychic cost for a sense of belonging. Such costliness can result in the equally unsatisfactory outcome of being the un-embraceable *other*. Increasingly, Africana people in China must find a mid-course, the place of in-between-ness that allows for some affirmation of belonging and a degree of embracing of difference; of them being *other*.

Such a position does come with emotional costs, as many Africana people also face constraints on self-development that are a legacy from home or a function of living in China. They must mourn some of the lost pleasures of the past and resist the temptation to retreat into nostalgia or mindless consumption. The outsider status with its considerable distance can generate feelings of loneliness, as many Africana persons often lack many available peers or substantive relationships with Chinese persons. To their Chinese hosts, the foreigners represent difference and change, which are often a threat to tradition and therefore a perceived threat to the host country's cultural stability. Exacerbating the foreigners' possible isolation is their reluctance to accept constraints that limit a sense of independence, thereby leaving them with relatively few sources of validation.

Some Africana workers are able to establish a network of the like-minded, exemplified by many Africana professionals in Shanghai who are in networks that are wide but shallow. Such networks are good at addressing technical needs but less robust on speaking to socio-emotional concerns, as those requires more substantive and enduring relationships than are typical for cosmopolitans with their peripatetic lifestyles. Given their self-positioning outside of traditional groups, this means that the primary identity they often gravitate to is that of their career identity, which is often at the cost of limiting socio-emotional growth.

Membership in these intellectually oriented groups is based on being skilled, and, therefore, they place high demands on themselves to be accepted as members of the meritocracy (Strenger, 2016). This is in contrast to the Africana trading communities of southern China, where kinship ties are more evident but not without their own ambivalences, given the necessary accommodation to market forces. The merit-oriented groups are always preoccupied with performance, and this is anxiety-provoking to workers given their lack of embedment in a community where membership is also based on socio-emotional factors, not simply the cold calculus of productivity. This puts them on a treadmill of performing to meet ever-increasing standards. Performance is all that matters, and they are therefore impatient with process and traditions that hamper creativity and productivity (Strenger, 2016). They are thus drawn to places and institutions that minimize such impediments; places that yearn for their talents, appeal to their narcissism, and assuage their ego ideals. Such individuals are often heavily invested in distancing from smothering traditions and archaic processes.

Time is not the friend of individuals such as Africana persons in China, who are in these positions of permanent transition and who might luxuriate in their sense of *otherness*. Although they derive considerable pleasure and benefits from their outsider status, they must cope with frustration and anxiety resulting from unethical constraints and high levels of uncertainty, as well as their indifference to building community. For foreign workers such as the Africana ones in China, the ambivalence generated from being in a permanent state of in-between-ness requires them to develop adequate coping strategies. Those who are emotionally supple and intellectually astute are able to achieve the intellectual mobility they lacked at home and also some degree of the social and emotional gratifications necessary for a rounded sense of well-being in China. Stalking them, however, is always the sense of an irreducible degree of exclusion that, upon reflection, while keenly felt in China, originates in a comparable sense of being an outsider at home. In-between-ness becomes a permanent state of being accompanied by ambivalence and the need to develop adaptive coping strategies.

Possibilities

Positive recognition is derived from people such as fellow countrymen, ethnic peers, and Chinese individuals with whom Africana persons have cultivated a substantive relationship and with whom they share deep humanistic values.

Such work speaks to the emergence of hybrid aspects of the self that, because of their in-between-ness, cannot be easily classified. Such individuals must tolerate the periodic self-questioning as to who they are. These hybridities facilitate the recognition and enjoyment of the pleasures of otherness. The adaptive engagement of otherness animates individuals and affirms their reason for being. To the degree that there is engagement and dialogue, there is then the possibility of mutual recognition and the awareness of the particularity, difference, and commonality with other:

> Far better to open yourself to the irruption of the other: not just into your life, but into the order of your world. Just for a moment did you not feel that a door had opened into another world, not just into the hallway of your apartment building but into infinity?
>
> (Alford, 2002, p. 14)

A positive recognition of self as other is derived from multiple sources, an important one being the intellectual skill sets brought to, or further developed from being in, China. Such recognition of difference validates an otherness that garners admiration and material benefits for the Africana person. This is evident among astute traders, canny businesspersons, and gifted teachers. The skills of Africana workers are enhanced by the refreshing perspectives that they develop, given their immersion in difference and their bias to be curious and to be reflective.

They will derive pleasure from the unique perspectives they have and their capacity to be surprised. The Africana worker's increased capacity to explore and to be spontaneous allows for exhilarating re-acquaintance with heretofore marginalized aspects of the self and discovery of new forms of self-awareness and expression.

Places such as China struggle with a conundrum in that there is a desire for social spaces that facilitates certain market-oriented forms of creativity. At the same time, there are often attempts to actively constrain creative individuals' who deploy their skills to advocate for human rights. Africana workers, among others who have sought to engage in advocacy, elicit a sharp and negative response from the state.

The healthy life requires social engagement, and with such responsibility comes what Alford (2002) refers to as "persecuted subjectivity"; the only way in which subjectivity may be known is as "the prosecution of the narcissism of the I" (pp. 16–17). Ideally, one is always subject to this "good violence," this ethical persecution and curb on narcissism. Such engagement should ideally be informed by the sentiments of sympathy and empathy; constraints should be exercised in the context of caring relationships where one strives to stay engaged and understand the other.

Therefore Africana workers in China, while committed to self-development, are also challenged to engage the otherness in which they are embedded and to manage the ambivalence generated by such work.

References

Adams, C. J. (2015). Structure and agency: Africana immigrants in China. *Journal of Pan African Studies*, *7*(10), 85–108.

Akhtar, S. (1995). A third individuation: Immigration, identity and the psychoanalytic process. *Journal of the American Psychoanalytic Association*, *43*(4), 1051–1084.

Alford, C. (2002). *Levinas, the Frankfurt School and psychoanalysis*. Middletown, CT: Wesleyan University Press.

Balogun, O. (2011). No necessary tradeoff: Context, life course, and social network identity information of second-generation Nigerians in the USA. *Ethnicities*, *11*(4), 436–466.

Bauman, Z. (1991). *Modernity and ambivalence*. London, UK: Polity Press.

Bauman, Z. (2001). Identity in the globalizing world. *Social Anthropology*, *9*(2), 121–129.

Beltsiou, J. (2016). Seeking home in the foreign: Otherness and immigration. In J. Beltsiou (Ed.), *Immigration in psychoanalysis* (pp. 89–108). New York, NY: Routledge.

Bodomo, A. (2012). *Africans in China*. Amherst, NY: Cambria Press.

Botticelli, S. (2004). The politics of relational psychoanalysis. *Psychoanalytic Dialogues*, *14*(5), 635–651.

Bromberg, P. (1996). Standing in the spaces: The multiplicity of self and the psychoanalytic relationship. *Contemporary Psychoanalysis*, *32*, 509–535.

Bureau of Labor Statistics. (2017a). Computer programmers. *Occupational Outlook Handbook, 2016–17 Edition*. Retrieved from www.bls.gov/ooh/computer-and-information-technology/computer-programmers.htm

Bureau of Labor Statistics. (2017b). Software developers. *Occupational Outlook Handbook, 2016–17 Edition*. Retrieved from www.bls.gov/ooh/computer-and-information-technology/software-developers.htm

Chun, A. (2009). On the geopolitics of identity. *Anthropological Theory*, *9*(3), 331–349.

Cisse, D. (2015). African traders in Yiwu: Their trade networks and their role in the distribution of "made in China" products in Africa. *Journal of Pan African Studies*, *7*(10), 44–64.

Conway, D. (2007). Caribbean transnational migration behavior: Reconceptualizing its "strategic flexibility." *Population, Space and Place*, *13*, 415–431.

Echeruo, M. (1999). An African diaspora: The ontological project. In I. Okpewho, C. Davies, & A. Mazrui (Eds.), *The African diaspora* (pp. 3–18). Bloomington, IN: Indiana University Press.

Elliot, A. (2002). *Psychoanalytic theory: An introduction* (2nd ed.). Durham, NC: Duke University Press.

Fanon, F. (1967). *Black skin, white masks*. New York, NY: Grove Press.

Freire, P. (2000). *Pedagogy of the oppressed*. New York, NY: Continuum.

Freud, S. (1961). *Civilization and its discontents*. London, UK: W. W. Norton & Co.

Frosh, S. (2013). Psychoanalysis, colonialism, racism. *Journal of Theoretical and Philosophical Psychology, 33*(3), 141–154.

Fuss, D. (1994). Interior colonies: Frantz Fanon and the politics of identification. *Diacritics, 24*(2/3), 19–42.

Gordon, L. (2000). *Existentia Africana: Understanding Africana existential thought*. New York, NY: Routledge.

Grinberg, L., & Grinberg, R. (1982). *Psychoanalytic perspectives on migration and exile*. New Haven, CT: Yale University Press.

Hall, S. (1990). Cultural identity and diaspora. In J. Rutherford (Ed.), *Identity, community, culture and difference* (pp. 222–237). London, UK: Lawrence & Wishart.

Hall, S. (2002). Political belonging in a world of multiple identities. In S. Vertovec & R. Cohen (Eds.), *Conceiving cosmopolitanism: Theory, context and practice* (pp. 25–32). New York, NY: Oxford University Press.

Haugen, H. (2012). Nigerians in China: A second state of immobility. *International Migration, 50*(2), 65–80.

Haugen, H., & Diederich, M. (2016a). Decision to leave home. Retrieved from https://uturnasia.com/2016/01/26/test/

Haugen, H., & Diederich, M. (2016b). From the Gambia to China. Retrieved from https://uturnasia.com/2016/01/25/test11/

Haugen, H., & Diederich, M. (2016c). Life in China. Retrieved from https://uturnasia.com/2016/01/24/test-1/

Haugen, H., & Diederich, M. (2016d). Getting out of China. Retrieved from https://uturnasia.com/2016/01/23/18/

Haugen, H., & Diederich, M. (2016e). Returning home. Retrieved from https://uturnasia.com/2016/01/22/returning-home/

Haugen, H., & Diederich, M. (2016f). Imagining a future. Retrieved from https://uturnasia.com/2016/01/20/aspirations/

Headley, C. (2011). George Lamming and the epistemology of exile: Ways of seeing, singularity and colonialism. In A. Bogues (Ed.), *The George Lamming reader: The aesthetics of decolonialisation* (pp. 287–310). Kingston, Jamaica: Ian Randle Publishers.

Hermans, H., & Dimaggio, G. (2007). Self, identity, and globalization in times of uncertainty: A dialogical analysis. *Review of General Psychology, 11*(1), 31–61.

Hopper, E. (2002). *The social unconscious: Selected papers*. London, UK: Jessica Kingsley.

Kipnis, A. (2007). Neoliberalism reified: Suzhi discourse and tropes of neoliberalism in the People's Republic of China. *Journal of the Royal Anthropological Institute, 13*, 383–400.

Levinas, E. (1985). *Ethics and infinity* (R. A. Cohen, Trans.). Pittsburgh, PA: Duquesne University Press.

McGowan, T. (2016). *Capitalism and desire*. New York, NY: Columbia University Press.

Menozzi, C. (2016). International migration report 2015. *The Department of Economic and Social Affairs of the United Nations Secretariat*. Retrieved from www.un.org/en/.../migration/.../migrationreport/.../MigrationReport 2015_Highlights.p

Mitchell, S. (1993). *Hope and dread in psychoanalysis*. New York, NY: Basic Books.

Nandy, A. (1998a). *Return from exile*. New Delhi: Oxford University Press.

Nandy, A. (1998b). The savage Freud: The first non-Western psychoanalyst and the politics of secret selves in colonial India. In *The savage, Freud and other essays on possible and retrievable selves* (pp. 81–144). In A. Nandy (Author) *Return from exile*. New Delhi: Oxford University Press.

Naujoks, D. (2010). Diasporic identities: Reflections on transnational belongings. *Diaspora Studies*, *3*(1), 1–21.

Scott, D. (2005). Stuart Hall's ethics. *Small Axe*, *17*(9), 1–16.

Strenger, C. (2013). The new cosmopolitans: Challenges and discontents. *Psychoanalytic Psychology*, *30*(2), 264–280.

Strenger, C. (2016). *Freud's legacy in the global era*. New York, NY: Routledge.

Walls, G. (2003). Toward a critical global analysis. *Psychoanalytic Dialogues*, *14*(5), 605–634.

Williams, H. (2016). A neocolonial warp of outmoded hierarchies, curricula and disciplinary technologies in Trinidad's educational system. *Critical Studies in Education*. Retrieved from http://dx.doi.org/10.1080/17508487.2016.1237982

Zhao, K. (2015). Stephon Marbury gains museum, and green card, in China. *New York Times*. Retrieved from www.nytimes.com/2015/12/24/world/asia/stephon-marbury-china-basketball.html?&moduleDetail=section-news-0&action=click&contentCollection=Pro%20Basketball%C2%AEion= Footer&module=MoreInSection&version=WhatsNext&contentID= WhatsNext&pgtype=article

3 Adaptive Ambivalence

Modernity and Ambivalence

Modernity might well be referred to as the age of ambivalence (Bauman, 1991; Freud, 1961) given the tension between the necessity support to facilitate the aspirations around individuation and agency and the constraints (some due to unethical policies such as resource withholding) placed on those aspirations. To make matters more complex, all of this occurs within a larger context of capitalist rapaciousness and the retreat of the protective state. Ambivalence is therefore a feature of such strivings given the need to also accept, however reluctantly, that opportunities for self-improvement exist alongside constraints on their pursuit.

Many Africana people in China are often embedded in diverse and well-resourced networks that provide the support necessary for them to develop adaptive ways of managing the vicissitudes that come with relating and working (Adams, 2015). Informed by a sense of the home culture's perspectives and other experiences prior to coming to China, they develop, over time a psychosocial perspective that has an unblinking view of opportunity and accompanying constraint. This position of adaptive ambivalence toward both home and host countries is informed by the need to wrestle with an existential dilemma: They have substantive reasons to be attracted to home and to China, alongside equally substantive dissatisfactions with both. Ideally, from a position of adaptive ambivalence, over time they develop the psychological capacities to neither idealize nor disparage either of these psychological bases in pursuit of self-development and self-growth. One subject illustrated his ambivalence when he spoke of his love for his home country along with the realization that it offered few opportunities for substantive professional growth and the attendant improvement in self-worth. China, by contrast, was exciting, as he could develop his creative skills there, be well paid, travel frequently, and have diverse, if not always substantial, friendships. He also celebrated an evolution of himself that was confident and assertive, and celebrated his sense of Blackness and the broadening of his worldview.

Alongside this were feelings of loneliness, being subjected to racism, and the realization that he would never be fully accepted into Chinese society. He has demonstrated a psychological stance that I am classifying as *adaptive ambivalence*: being attuned to and able to manage in a healthy way the ambivalence that arises from having to navigate both opportunities and constraints with regard to self-development in whatever place he resides. While pleased with a sense of accomplishment, this positive feeling sits alongside a sense of a difficult-to-define unease that in its benign form is experienced as restlessness and a fuel for curiosity that allows for experiencing refreshing perspectives. At its worst, there is a sense of not quite belonging wherever they are and wishing that it were not so, and at the same time not being able to articulate what would adequately assuage such a lack.

This is what Said (1993) and Conway (2007) refer to as a state of "in-between-ness," a sense of wanting to be situated firmly in a given psychosocial space, but instead being on the periphery of those spaces, in this case between home and host country. This is complimented by Bhabha, who situates such a psychic space as "in-between the claims of the pasts and the needs of the future" (Bhabha, 1994, p. 219)

This bias toward a position of ambivalence often has its origins in the home country, where substantive structural constraints on personal development, alongside familial contretemps, are often in tension with a sense of being embedded in a community that loves and strives to validate its members as being special (Beltsiou, 2016; Said, 1993).

This ambivalence is heightened by the awareness of the psychosocial advantages and costs of living in the host culture. Many Africana workers are able to attain high levels of what in China is referred to as *suzhi* (Hairong, 2003): the ability to improve their capabilities and status, especially with regard to intellectual growth and material gain. *Suzhi* is, however, twinned to *chiku* (Hairong, 2003), or eating bitterness, which is the necessity for the individual to accept structurally imposed limits on aspirations in areas such as advocating for rights. This ambivalence is informed by a corresponding ambivalence within Chinese culture where, in the pursuit of national development, there is a desire for creative foreign workers alongside antipathy toward them and the difference they represent.

Vignette: Wei Wei

About Wei Wei

Wei Wei is a curious and perceptive 31-year-old relocation specialist from southern Africa with a postgraduate degree in international relations. She has lived all over the world starting at an early age, and she refers to herself as belonging to a class of "third-culture kids," having lived in Europe, South America, the Caribbean, and southern Africa. She has lived in Shanghai for the past 6 years with her husband and her 1-year-old son. Wei Wei is fluent and literate in Chinese: "I speak the language, I dream in Chinese," she says. At the same time, she has concerns about the quality of the physical environment in China and the limited educational facilities available to her child. Wei Wei also feels that despite her fluency in Chinese, she is still perceived as an outsider and must be vigilant about being discriminated against and exploited, especially when engaging in business transactions. Wei Wei illustrated this risk for a foreigner transacting business in China: She spoke in Chinese on the phone to negotiate a fee for some work to be done in her apartment, and then later the price was increased when the contractor realized she was a foreigner.

Wei Wei's experiences capture the core of adaptive ambivalence; even as she celebrates her successes, she must be mindful of the need to be vigilant and acceptance of the sense of only partial inclusion.

Shifting Sense of Home

Wei Wei was attracted to the allure of China, perceiving it as intriguingly different from her other cultural locales. Her notion of home is fluid given her upbringing, and she defines it as both wherever her mother resides and also wherever she, her husband, and her child reside. She is clear that China will never be their permanent home.

Pride vs. Need to Be Vigilant

Wei Wei is noted in Shanghai for her building of a Black community that is inclusive and sensitive to women's issues. These efforts validate her Blackness and create a safe space for other Black persons, especially women in Shanghai:

> My husband got frustrated with the "Spot the Black person" experience when he was out and about. I went to the fabric market and I saw a Black man from Zimbabwe and another from France. I decided to form a group and invited people to my house, but I did not expect 16 people to turn up. I felt loved.

She has also facilitated regular meetings of a group for Black women and hosts an annual Thanksgiving dinner. Being in China has reaffirmed her positive sense of Blackness:

> I always loved my Blackness as I grew up in a home where Black was beautiful. This is a good time to be Black as since Obama came to power everyone loves Blackness. I can do so much good as they

> do not know Blackness. While the image of Blackness in Shanghai is not too bad, it is very difficult in Guangzhou.

Wei Wei, as a dark-skinned Africana woman, is quite attuned to the privileging of Whiteness in Chinese culture: "They associate paleness of skin with wealth and high status. If you are a cosmetics company, you must have a skin whitening product." At the same time, the apparent admiration of Whiteness is subjected to an important caveat: "Idolizing Whites does not mean they like them. Some vendors will say, I like you, but I do not like Whites. We have all suffered under the Whites," she says. Whiteness is used here to indicate an admiration of skin shade and is not necessarily linked to the unthoughtful admiration of the cultural attributes of White persons of European heritage. This apparent bounded racial privileging by some Chinese people resonates with some entitled White males, who are therefore made uncomfortable by Wei Wei's assertion of her Blackness and by her group facilitating activities:

> White men especially do not understand the need for a support system. I do not want to be seen as the stereotype, the angry Black woman. We must have our act together, we must be strong. You want to cry in a safe place.

Wei-Wei feels a sense of having grown psychological in China, in ways not possible in the West:

> I have grown more confident. It feels so foreign without my mother. I really can do anything; I can make anything work. I also feel more empowered. Being in China gives you a sense of worth. Here I know the residents and I have formed relationships; there is a sense of pride. That would not have happened in the United States or Europe; there you do not make a difference. Here, you can talk across status boundaries.

Given her sense of pride alongside her sense of the necessity to be vigilant, Wei Wei exemplifies one presentation of a stance of adaptive ambivalence.

Difficulty Belonging vs. Forming Close Friendships

Wei Wei noted that the Chinese can be quite flexible if one does not put them in a position where taking a different approach would cause them to lose face. Spontaneity is therefore difficult to elicit given the reluctance to casually voice perspectives that appear to challenge traditional ways of doing things: "If it is not written on paper, they are not going to do it. Do not ask them to go off script. Do not ask them to think," says Wei Wei.

To Wei Wei, this emphasis on tradition presents challenges in dealing with foreigners. While wary toward foreigners, including Blacks, Wei Wei portrays the Chinese more as being ignorant about racial and ethnic differences than as being xenophobic and uniformly racist toward Africana persons in China: "They are very cautious with foreigners. This was a closed society for a very long time. So there are degrees of being let in. It is a very gradual process."

Wei Wei goes on to give an interesting gender twist:

> [T]hey are curious but not necessarily hostile toward my Blackness. So lots of whispering, they do not quite know what to do with us, especially women. They see a lot more Black men than Black women; they take their model of Blacks from American television so they whisper that my husband is an NBA star.

Despite these cultural challenges, Wei Wei has developed close and gratifying relationships with some Chinese persons. She portrays them as being very utilitarian in their approach to relationships and argues that success comes from being persistent in a low-key manner. Wei Wei spent hours socializing with the owner of a nail salon and, in the process, improving her Chinese fluency skills, her perspectives on the culture, and being known as an individual.

> People are not going to bother with you if they think you are going to be staying for only a short time. My best friend is a Chinese woman. I would go to her store and really culture a relationship with her. She told me she was pregnant before she told her husband.

Brief Analysis

Wei Wei is quite attuned to the pleasures and costs of being a dark-skinned Africana woman in China and has further honed adaptive ways of managing the ambivalence it re-animates within her. She has a strong and diverse support group that allows her to avoid making facile and unthoughtful comments with regard to the strengths and challenges that both Chinese and Africana persons must manage in their dealings with each other. Crucial for adaptive functioning, as demonstrated by Wei Wei, is the ability to manage the tension between the legacy of culture in terms of its influence on self-making and the capacity to be reflective and chart a relatively autonomous path, influenced but not determined by culture. Wei Wei is also able to have a clear-eyed view of the constraints she faces with regard to self-development and to constantly assess them relative to the opportunities that China offers. Adequately managing the tension between cost and opportunity is the heart of doing adaptive ambivalence.

Origins of Ambivalence

Bauman (1991) and Freud (1961) both argue for ambivalence being a central feature of the modern condition, resulting in individuals being somewhat constrained in their attempts to be autonomous as the cost of belonging to a group that strives to minimize conflict and promote harmony. This inevitably generates an irreducible degree of conflict, with the individual striving to be spontaneous, pleasure-seeking, and unfettered, while at the same time requiring group support in the form of recognition, protection, and facilitating skill acquisition. The group in the form of family, community, or administrative state is ambivalent about individuality, as while it is a source of creativity and productivity, in its most unfettered form it is a threat to the harmony and integrity of the group. The individual, by the same token, treasures the idea of the pursuit of curiosity and pleasure but can only do so for any sustained period and in a relatively safe way in the context of group support. The outcome is ambivalence at both the level of the individual and the group, manifested as each having mixed feelings toward the other, (Freud, 1961).

Further feeding the ambivalence is the fact that the individual's primordial urges are often targeted by capitalism, resulting in the individual being seduced into privileging the gratification of the primitive at the often considerable cost of being reflective, self-disciplined, and altruistic. Attempts to effectively manage this tension are often less than successful given the absence of any definitive guidance, including that of a well-functioning ethical compass. Ambivalence becomes the default position given uncertainty, attraction, and risk.

Such an outcome is reflective of Russell's (1990) approach to ambivalence, which he defines as uncertainty given two choices, both of which are valid, equally attractive, and on a continuum as opposed to being binary. So, for example, it is not unusual when speaking to Africana persons in China to hear them speak about its attractions. Kristina, a former bank executive, observed:

> This is the cockpit of the world. This is an investment in my future. I am learning Chinese and it will pay off for me, between the Chinese [competency] and the [completed] book. This is a front seat on the global stage. To keep sharp and competitive you have to be here.

These are not unconditional attractions, as while both sites are attractive, they are also perceived as having mirror-like shortcomings. China is admired relative to home given the availability of the pleasures that can be gratified through the pursuit of intellectual and economic opportunities, that are scarce at home. The home country is liked because of the emotional gratifications to be derived from attachments to family and community and the sense of being recognized and embraced, features that are less available in Chinese cultural spaces. The sites are neither fully embraced nor totally rejected, hence the ambivalence. Adding complexity to the psychodynamics of recognition in the host country, is China's marked ambivalence toward foreigners, who, while admired for their intellectual skills or business acumen, are viewed warily as representative of cultural difference.

Max Weber's perspective on ambivalence was that it had its roots in the absence of a strong sense of ethics; such ethics, while crucial for healthy life, was difficult in modern conditions (Smart, 1999).

> For Weber, prevailing conditions meant disenchantment, rationalization, and discipline, conditions that rendered social conditions impersonal and thereby increasingly inaccessible to ethical interpretation. It is the marginalization or the disfiguring of face-to-face ethical relations that Weber identifies as the most significant consequence of modern processes of rationalization.
>
> (Smart, 1999, p. 3)

Without such an ethics, not only are relations impoverished, but there is the risk of the individual embracing the primitive, thereby triggering a harsh counter-response by the group in an attempt to limit the destabilization that occurs when normative, if not always ethical, attachments are weakened. In such ethically challenged settings, there is the seduction of the primitive, a wish for order, low social trust, and a resulting heightened ambivalence toward any given course of action. One consistent theme among the sample of Africana persons in China who I interviewed was the ethical challenges they faced in their business transactions in China, a sense of having to be always vigilant less they be exploited. This concern was not limited to Chinese individuals and institutions but often included ethnic kin and other foreigners in China.

There is an irreducible tension between the group's demand for harmony and the individual's pursuit of pleasure. An example of an extreme manifestation of this tension is in relation to migration issues: the refusal of Japan to allow substantial in-migration to offset the steep decline in its population due to low reproduction rates and an increasingly elderly population (Kashiwazaki & Akaha, 2006; Oishi, 2012). This ambivalence toward cultural difference is also reflected in China's policy of rarely granting permanent residence status alongside its insistence that most foreigners are granted only 1-year visas, no matter how long they have resided in China. Such wariness is not limited to Asia, as is evident in the immigration policies of the United Kingdom, among others. It would seem that the wariness toward difference and positive change, as manifested by the outsider and individuality, sometimes trumps the threat of group decline.

Paradoxically, the dominant group, with its questionable adoption of neoliberalism, will use state-sanctioned authority to extract work while at the same time constraining the degree of agency individuals are able to exercise and the amount of pleasure they derive from the work (Crouch, 2016; Foster, 2016; McGowan, 2016). For many Africana persons who have historically worked under such conditions and those who currently labor with meager results, the dominant group is viewed with a high degree of ambivalence. Many will seek to leave and join groups where they experience relatively fewer restrictions on agency and greater degrees of gratification (Senior, 2014; Wilkerson, 2010). Such motives are what drives many of the reasons for migrating. At the same time, there is a sense that the pressures to adjust to the demands of the group increase the level of ambivalence, while at the same time an individual's need to feel more accepted and have pleasurable experiences is largely unmet (Kleinman et al., 2011; Smart, 1999).

A second paradox is that given that human aggression and the pursuit of pleasure cannot be completely eliminated, invariably the group generates products—especially under capitalist regimes—that appeal to pleasure and aggression, and therefore are unwittingly complicit in destabilizing the group. The offering of cheap consumer products in the context of low wages requires long working hours by the individual, which reduces the time available for intimacy, family life, and community building. These offerings generally appeal to an often shallow self-interest, not to substantive self-growth or to group harmony. In China, the pursuit of the material is widely encouraged but has led to a fraying of the social net (Blumenthal & Hsiao, 2005; Kleinman et al., 2011) and to environmental degradation (Wong, 2015). These are a reflection of a marginalization of the ethical informed attention to the common good.

Another consequence of this over-management of the individual's pursuit of pleasure is a reduction in risk taking. A risk-averse individual often keeps a tight rein on curiosity and *jouissance*, with an attendant reluctance to challenge the hegemony of tradition, stasis, and subordination. One result of this, as noted by Freud (1961); Fanon (1967); and Freire (2000), among others, is that the prohibitions of the group can dominate the thoughts and influence the behavior of the individual. This is especially risky for subordinated groups, such as those found in some Africana communities, where what are thought to be appropriate ways of thinking and behaving represent the priorities of the dominant group to the detriment of the individual (Adams, 2007). There is reluctance on the part of some Africana individuals to challenge the status quo, and this leads to a need for greater self-discipline to contain frustration and anger. It also can lead to more risk-aversive behaviors and higher levels of ambivalence.

Such an outcome results when the individual focuses on being acquisitive and therefore is overly invested in the material aspects of the world

(Fromm, 1976). The self that is overly attuned to consume shies away from being reflective, for fear of the anxiety that will be experienced at the thought of restraining the pursuit of shallow pleasures. The task of living a less materialistically oriented life in pursuit of a difficult-to-define and elusive authenticity is daunting for many. Such a thrust might well put individuals in conflict with the group, should they demand structural changes to facilitate their attempts at authentic and ethical self-development.

Too harsh a disciplinary stance by the group could trigger nihilistic behaviors by the individual. By contrast, any reasonable accommodation leaves individuals to some degree ambivalent as they are attracted to the pleasures of the primitive, but must also accept some hopefully ethically informed, group-imposed constraints that counterbalance the benefits of the agency they afford. The individual's life course can be seen, to some degree, as a measure of how she or he manages this existential ambivalence.

Modern individuals must cope with being the managers of their moral compasses and the ethical behaviors that result from such a perspective. This task is reflective of a shift in the responsibility for thinking about how to live an ethical life. Rules that were once primarily mandated by institutions are now generated by the individual. This is both exciting and daunting for, among others, Africana individuals in China must adopt a robust reflective capacity that allows them to effectively manage the ambivalences arising from being socialized in one ambiguous moral landscape, in the home country, while living in another, namely China.

Contemporary Perspectives on Ambivalence: A Critique of Modernity as Purely Dystopian

As noted earlier by Weber and also by Foucault, there is a sense of the marginalization of the ethical from the public sphere, with the responsibility for the moral being placed on the individual (Joas, 2013). Such a shift weakens the affective ties between the institution and the individual, and this in turn lessens the capacity of the institution to either provide a moral framework or to demand ethical behavior from the individual (Foster, 2016).This dystopian turn does not go uncontested, and Joas (2013) argues that despite the attempt at marginalization, one can observe an ethical mobilization. This places an emphasis on the sacred within the individual and the attendant respect for human dignity and rights advocacy:

> I propose that we understand the belief in human rights and universal human dignity as the result of a specific process of sacralization—a process in which every single human being has increasingly, and

> with ever-increasing motivational and sensitizing effects, been viewed as sacred, and this understanding has been institutionalized in law.
>
> (p. 5)

This sense of the individual as sacred is a source of enhanced agency for individuals who are increasingly expected to be entrepreneurs of the self, within the context of an institutional framework that they might well have to advocate for. At the same time, this sacralization of the self feeds the ambivalence inherent in the modern condition, as the individual must rely more on a self that is conflicted about being ethical.

In the quest for individuals to manage moral ambiguity and the attendant risk of unethical behavior, Joas (2013) argues for the importance of being thoughtful about the full range of experiences we have in the process of living our lives, as it is these experiences that are the midwife of values that shape how we define ourselves. On this issue, Joas addresses the need for the reflective individual to contemplate both past and present: "This is not a matter of an alternative between a historical or present-day orientation; instead, gaining a historically grounded understanding of the present helps solve contemporary orientational problems" (p. 124).

For many Africana persons coming from countries with a legacy of colonialism, neocolonialism, ethnic, and racial discrimination, such insight is crucial as they seek to assert an ethically informed agency in China. Home countries were often characterized by a state that was often indifferent to ethical norms of conduct and respected few rights of the individual. Such behavior often had its origins in a capitalist ideology that viewed the individual as an enslaved person whose surplus productivity was purloined by rentiers who controlled the mechanisms of power. For many, the alternate indigenous institutions of power, while morally informed, were often highly paternalistic and rigid, leaving scant room for individuality and rights advocacy. The individual was either exploited by one group or subject to the harsh disciplinary regimes of the other. Joas (2013) notes the culturally informed quality of values, as a result of which many Africana persons, among others struggle with being ethical guided individuals.

So, for many Africana persons, home is a source of oppression given a history of the subordination of the individual. Fromm (1976); Fanon (1967); and Khanna (2003) and others have argued that some cultural configurations can lead to various forms of psychopathology, individual ways of developing that distort desire, leave conflict unresolved, and limit agency.

While home is also a site of pleasure with regard to intimacy and aesthetics, given its often harsh and unethical governance structures, it is also a site of restriction and immobility. The skills developed at home, alongside the limits of home, are internalized and accompany migrants as they go abroad in search of a growth-facilitating space.

The pre-migratory experience generates not only ambivalence about home, but also the risk of a legacy of immobility that can be exacerbated in China due to the lack of marketable capabilities and lack of access to facilitating networks. Haugen (2012), in her seminal work on Africana traders in southern China, notes the degree of immobility experienced and its links to home:

> For some of my informants, the frustrations over immobility and the desire to leave Nigeria had been intensified by personal problems, such as coercion into an undesired marriage, conflicts with senior family members or frustrated professional ambitions. Such idiosyncratic events can intensify the search for migration opportunities and make potential migrants more inclined to head for less desirable destinations.
>
> (p. 71)

Thus the immobility immigrants internalize and carry with them from their home countries can sometimes be exacerbated by structural and practical factors in their new countries of residence. These in turn can add yet more layers of immobility or can put them at a disadvantage to begin with in terms of influencing such basic decisions as to their choice of destination.

Thus in China, among other increasingly neoliberal settings, the moral self is increasingly in tension with the enterprising self. To effectively manage this requires a degree of vigilance and thoughtfulness to be both ethical and successful. Africana workers speak to being judicious as to when to be tolerant about rule violations and when to take a firm stance. Some, such as the businessmen in Yiwu or the community leaders in Guangzhou, seek, with varying degrees of success, to negotiate for fair administrative rulings.

Others have noted the need for vigilance with kin from home who seek to exploit their generosity or ethnic kin who act unethically in business dealings. Such actions speak to the necessity of balancing self-protection and progress with moral action, requiring more than a passing familiarity with understanding similarity within difference and difference that is truly different. Such an examination facilitates the expansion of ethical and gratifying ways of being in the world. Yet many Africana persons in China struggle with the felt need to consistently act in ethical ways.

The skepticism of modernity and its emphasis on the contingent nature of life tend to overlook the fact that the individual, especially in dialogue with others, is an influential contingent factor. The individual is more than simply an anxious and ambivalent respondent to other contingent factors. So, the reflective individual, in dialogue with others, influences the decision as to how to act in a given environment of uncertainty (Hermans & Dimaggio, 2007). While this process is at times unconscious, it has a historical foundation that influences how the individual acts, as against adherence to some abstract criteria as to how to act in the world (Joas, 2013). This approach emphasizes individuals' history and their capacity to reflect and dialogue, so as to make them open to new approaches in the pursuit of goals. Wei Wei illustrated that not being a prisoner to her history and being open to new ideas and to engaging in dialogue with those who are different, has enabled her to thrive.

For some Africana traders, the challenge is managing the tendency of engaging in narrow, often unethical, and possibly antagonistic interactions with Chinese peers. Many spoke of being tempted to go beyond being ethically vigilant and to engaging in unscrupulous behavior. For the technocrats, the risk is an indifference to engaging with a diverse set of Chinese people, and many limit themselves to socializing only with English-speaking peers with a Western orientation. In both cases, there is no substantive dialogue with Chinese persons, so there is little opportunity to have one's perspective validated or to be challenged by a difference that might be really different. As a consequence, feelings of ambivalence are not assuaged given the paucity of positive experiences that are based on nurturing commonalities and exploring differences with a diverse range of Chinese persons.

The space within which the Africana person attempts to fulfill healthy desires also engenders ambivalence as it is often fraught with ethical challenges. That which might be desired might be seemingly innocuous but may be prohibited for ideological reasons. This is evident in China with regard to restraints on some forms of religious worship, gender, and sexual expression or community organizing. The ambivalence could be linked to a particular space because of its facilitatory and at the same time restrictive tendencies in relation to the various aspects of the desires of the individual.

So, as we have seen, for the modern individual, some degree of loss and constraint, alongside opportunity, are constant bedfellows. Part of loss is accepting that desire can never be completely assuaged, and that because of such limits on growth there is also a limit on self-expression (Khanna, 2003). To be in China is to be restrained about making any complaints about unethical aspects of the political system and also to mourn the realization that one will probably not be granted Chinese citizenship.

Loss, mourning, and melancholy are therefore inherent features of modern life, especially among individuals who have experienced structural oppression or who have left their homeland. The individual must come to terms with the need to accept the idea of both irretrievable loss and the possibility of reimagining and recreating the self. This intrapsychic tension can lead to a well-informed wish to have a greater say over narrating and interpreting one's life. The possibility of actually engaging in such work can become a reality, given that there is an increased sense not only of interpretive room, but also an awareness of prior, often unconscious but limiting interpretive models.

Africana people in pursuit of self-development are quite familiar with loss and with growth as they venture abroad. The gratifications of home and China, alongside their constraints, require the Africana worker to be vigilant with regard to opportunities for pleasure and the inevitability of being constrained. Implied here is that ambivalence is increasingly evident as a function of dis-embedding from the seemingly homogenous, familiar, and limiting and re-embedding in the seemingly heterogeneous with its differences and opportunities. In summary, a given individual is embedded in cultural settings that both gratify and frustrate self-strivings to some degree. Adaptive ways of managing the resultant ambivalence permit growth alongside some acceptance of limits, sufficient to avoid triggering intolerable ethical limitations, or disapproval from the group.

The Process of Adaptive Ambivalence

An adaptive approach to managing ambivalence holds in tension both the love and limits of home alongside the possibilities and constraints that exist within the host country. It facilitates the Africana person exploiting a space within which to pursue growth and to revel in a sense of agency and status that was not attainable at home. In China, many Africana people have enhanced their considerable intellectual skills and have been well remunerated by the marketplace. With the financial surpluses generated, they can delve further into self-discovery through travel, permitted spiritual exploration, and cultivating diverse cultural relationships. These activities reaffirm the self as being intelligent, curious, and effective. In addition, they re-animate long-frustrated feelings of healthy difference and individuality. There is a sense of perceiving the confident self as not unduly smothered by the suffocating love from home or the limits of its administrative structures. They enjoy the pleasures derived from the unique perspective afforded by the in-between space from which they view themselves, their home countries, and China. Gleanings from that place enrich their capacity to be creative and assertive and to effectively manage the irreducible need to at times eat bitterness, to accept limits; what the Chinese refer to as *chiku*.

The Africana individual is likely to be more creative and at the same time less complicit with the center by taking a dispassionate, if not jaundiced, view from the margin. Such a person can bring an unconventional point of view from such a self-positioning perspective, in contrast to those who are wedded to the normative and at ease within its embrace (Said, 1993). That in turn makes the individual more willing to take risks, comfortable with uncertainty: "the audacity of daring, and moving, moving, moving, representing change, not standing still" (Said, 1993, p. 124).

For some others, the desire may be to enjoy the pleasures of being uncommitted; they might revel in the ambivalence of in-between-ness. As Adorno noted, there is an attraction to and pleasure derived from a position of "not to be at home in one's home" (Said, 1993, p. 120). Ambivalence can therefore be animated by the pleasures derived from resisting the disciplinary moves of late modernity, with its emphasis on developing and deploying a rational and structured self that articulates and assuages desire in a conventional manner. This resonates with Said's happily unhappy motif where the desire is not necessarily to be understood or to be too settled and satisfied, a position that is helpful in managing ambivalence.

This speaks to issues of identity, ethics, and opportunities for Africana persons in China as there is also a greater appreciation of contingencies and processes that shape a given outcome (Said, 1993). This, I would argue, also makes some Africana persons in China potentially more aware of themselves as contingent actors with agency, but who must also eat bitterness as it occurs in the context of in-between-ness. From the position of such a double perspective, the individual is better able to be dispassionate, avoid fatalistic and essentialist thinking, and keep a tight rein on both cynicism and unbounded hope.

These substantive attributes strengthen the Africana individual's ability to manage the costliness of being a stranger in a foreign land. Liberated from a simplistic view of home as the place that satisfies all needs, the individual is able to tolerate the restraints on some aspects of self-development that are experienced in China. Africana individuals come to uneasy accommodation with the racial slights and the unethical business culture, and they are careful to curb the temptation to negatively homogenize and denigrate the Chinese persons that they may not know well due to language limitations. So, while they are wary given some antipathy toward them as "African" and as foreigners, they are sufficiently resilient, given their positive experiences, not to embrace a blanket dystopian view of China.

On a more intimate level, some of them cultivate diverse relationships as a buffer against a tendency to adopt a superior stance toward their own cultural perspectives and an inferior one to matters Chinese. Again, they end up in an in-between space and are able to sustain such a stance if supported by similarly like-minded peers. Such relationships also assuage to some degree the loss of the idea of a settled home. Said (1993) speaks to this sense of being restless and unsettled: "You can't go back to some earlier and perhaps more stable condition of being at home; and alas, you can never fully arrive, be at one with your new home or situation" (p. 117).

As we have seen, ambivalence is an inherent feature of being human given our desire to be unfettered along with our need for recognition, protection, attachments, and nurturance, and the ethical demands and constraints that come with that. As a consequence, conflict is an embedded feature within the self, and many argue that a stable and substantively gratified singular sense of self is an illusion in the modern world, in which the assumption of mastery and the attainment of certainty is impossible (Mitchell, 1993). The challenge for the individual is to seek new ways of understanding and managing desire, while at the same time managing the sense of ultimate futility, the realization that given the contingent nature of our lives, there is no grand plan, and that to some degree we will always be ambivalent and therefore dissatisfied. As such, the awareness of the multiple layers of ambivalence that are part of being human in the modern world and that can be multiplied for foreigners is the beginning of adaptively managing that very same ambivalence.

Central to adaptive ambivalence is that, for the Africana person in China, among others, is the realization of the bounded and increasingly questionable definition and achievability of the good life. They will orient instead to a growing awareness of its precariousness and the highly contingent pursuit of well-being. Adaptive ambivalence is therefore fueled by a felt history of both constraint and possibility wherever individuals are located as they are embedded within a larger psychosocial context of unresolvable discontent with modernity and civilization. Therefore, there is some degree of ontological resistance to assimilating wherever they reside, given a skeptical view of state and increasingly, market-mediated experiences of belonging. The individual must always reflect on the pursuit of that which is desired but was once forbidden or exercising autonomy where there was once dependency. This is conflict-ridden work with the ever-present risk of stasis and regression alongside the possibility of growth.

Ambivalence and Migration

I am challenging the traditional model of the psychic response to migration as that of being an inevitably and predominantly traumatic experience that requires mourning and relinquishing the investment in the original and un-conflicted internalizations of the experiences of home (Grinberg & Grinberg, 1982). While the decision to leave home can be psychologically painful, it is not necessarily traumatic, nor is it necessarily irreversible. Some forms of contemporary migration encompass pain in leaving and pleasures to be derived in going to a host country, and the realistic possibility of eventual return.

In the traditional model, the often reluctantly migrating individual is fleeing, never to return, and must assimilate into the new culture that is viewed as both benign and immutable toward the immigrant. To the degree that traditional immigrants are melancholic or resistant, they are compromising the possibility of coming to terms with the past and reimaging a more promising future. To the degree that the literature on immigrants insists on viewing the migration experience as unilaterally loss-oriented in relation to leaving home, we do a disservice to truth in ignoring the range and complexity of responses different people may experience. Further, ignoring a more complex experience of migration denies immigrants and those who work on the issue of migration the chance to identify and expand upon many generative and positive opportunities. I argue that some individuals who voluntarily leave their home countries adopt an ambivalent stance toward both home and toward the host country that can never be resolved but that can be managed adaptively.

For some immigrants, consciously adopting a stance of ambivalence is aided by the fact that the individual is not traumatized by leaving and has not renounced the possibility of return. I am also noting that being the other abroad comes with certain gratifications that inevitably exist in tension with a sense of in-between-ness and an occasional related irascibility (Conway, 2007; Lamming, 1984; Said, 1993). As an extension of this sense of ambivalence about location, my perspective also highlights the fact that Africana individuals may choose not to adopt an immigrant sensibility and may reject the expectation others may have of them of assimilating into Chinese society—especially given the cultural resistance and administrative obstacles to doing so. In addition, the immigrant might find pleasure in this particular form of otherness (Said, 1993).

Ambivalence and Community

Community can be thought of as a psychological and social space that addresses the individual's need for recognition and a sense of belonging to the group. It encompasses a space that facilitates strong emotional ties and reciprocity, in addition to benefits and rights (Berlant, 2011). Smart (1999) notes that all ethics are grounded in the interpersonal, which in turn requires a stable community to focus on, what Levinas (1985) refers to as "being for another" (p. 96), which is the bedrock of all ethics. Communities are ideally ethical, nurturing, and protective spaces arising from interdependent and enduring relationships. More often than not, the sense of belonging is often quite enduring, which is noteworthy given the fact that the community is not always able to adequately address the individual's needs in terms of providing resources and enforcing rights. Often what is provided can be emotionally quite costly, as the family can be materially and emotionally impoverished and inadequate to meet reasonable and vital demands for nurturance, protection, and the facilitation of aspirations. The group, through granting recognition and addressing the individual's need to belong, validates core components of the self, but at the same time, it is a source of ambivalence given the group's limited ability or willingness to facilitate substantive self-growth and autonomy.

Exacerbating the nature and quality of attachments to the community is the modernist shift from the group to the individual as the basic unit of modern Western culture. Contributing to this has been the enlightenment project with its emphasis on rationality and rights (Hampson, 1990), alongside the increasing use of technology as a handmaiden of increased and less costly agency. This shift has two important consequences in the meaning of the relationship between the individual and the community. First, the individual is less inclined to unquestionably accept the group's ideological dictates and its constraints on imagination, aspirations, and behavior (Bauman, 1991). A second consequence is the retreat of the community in the form of the state from being a source of nurturance and protection of the individual, as was its traditional role. It is no longer the institution that speaks to transcendence and to ethics, as those tasks have been shifted to the individual (Joas, 2013; Smart, 1999).

These shifts offer the individual the opportunity, in dialogue with others, of developing an ethically informed self and of assisting others, two phenomena that support attempts to create vibrant community. Individuals, however, must struggle with two risks, which inevitably leave them in a position of ambivalence (Hermans & Dimaggio, 2007). First, as noted earlier, they are not fully committed to being ethical beings, given their inherent narcissism and attraction to the primordial, hence their ambivalence about themselves. Second, the community in which they are embedded carries its own ambivalence about them given their capacity to disrupt. As a consequence, while the group may not nurture them as much as they would like, in late modernity, individuals will also be subject to high degrees of surveillance and possible harsh responses, especially if they call into question the ethical shortcomings of the community, as is often the case in China and in the home country. This yet further exacerbates the individual's own ambivalence about the community.

For some individuals, the shift to themselves as relatively self-absorbed and autonomous agents preoccupied with self-development might marginalize them from group obligations and constraints. Such a self is at best reduced to acts of private self-development or at worst into dissolute behaviors in a capitalistically seductive culture with a focus on consumption and the presentation of a false self (Strenger, 2016). The combination of ambivalence about community and about a sense of ethics that is relational rather than hierarchal often leaves the modern individual struggling with the question of how to balance self-needs with community demands. Feeding this uncertainty is the complexity of the modern group, which is a conglomeration of different subgroupings often with weak commonalities based on the narrow and often conflictual self-interests of its members. These conflictual demands occur in the larger context of the hegemony of neoliberal economic and political mandates that require subordination to market discipline and demand, regardless of how people define themselves.

As Berlant (2011) notes:

> There, there is no room to make a distinction among political, economic, and affective forms of existence, because the institutions of intimacy that constitute the everyday environments of the social are only viscerally but actually, as we know, intricately and dynamically related to all sorts of institutional, economic, historical, and symbolic dynamics.
>
> (p. 168)

In such settings, volatility is the norm, attachments are always under threat, and solidarity is at best tenuous and highly conditional (Smart, 1999). Yet the individual needs to belong and needs to feel recognized and therefore maintain affiliations, no matter how weakly and ambivalently. The risk here is that given how dissatisfying the normative can be, given the need to attach and be recognized, the individual might do so under any conditions, including those that are exploitive, in the hope that the attachment, no matter how emotionally costly and tenuous, is not broken (Berlant, 2011).

The Africana people I interviewed reported that Chinese people often perceive Africana people in China as a homogenous African grouping. They must accept such an ascription, especially when advocating for rights with the Chinese, irrespective of their national origins. For some, this can be emotionally costly, as is the case when, for example, a Guinean must find solidarity with a Nigerian, someone who belongs to a group she perceives with antipathy given experiences of being exploited by some of them in business transactions. Yet this Nigerian might be able to successfully advocate on her behalf with the Chinese authorities. In such cases, the individual struggles with the tension between distinct self-assertions and the need to subordinate them to a weakly held group identity so as to hopefully have her interests effectively addressed. For many Africana persons in China, that is the very reason they left home, questioning whether deferring to community mandates, especially in relation to family or the larger public good, was in their best interests. Many Africana individuals report a history of a style of relating in the home country that was often disingenuous or even injurious, bankrupting or thwarting self-interests with no commensurate pay off or compensation.

To the degree that community supports the rights of its members to be different, that can fragment community as people seek to establish their own rights community, with a narcissistic emphasis on difference. Community therefore has tenuous ties in this Baumanian "acceptance of the heterogeneity of dissensions" (Smart, 1999, p. 184). There is scant space for such Africana heterogeneity in China, with its emphasis on an imposed homogeneity that reflects the worldview of the ruling majority and seeks to severely constrain, if not obliterate, substantive cultural difference (Zang, 2015).

In a Chinese context, the expectation that the individual will become an ethical actor in the absence or reduced role of the state, while laudable, is daunting in the short to moderate run. The individual, as noted earlier, is ambivalent about being ethical, given the constraints it places on the pursuit of pleasure and exercise of aggression. Smart (1999) notes that while Levinas (1985) places emphasis on the task of the ethical individual to "be for another," Caputo (in Smart, 1999) asserts that this would be an unrealistically high standard to meet given our narcissistic nature and the need for to be recognized as having acted for another. Given also the absence of any agreed-upon foundational ethic, such actions could be risky, in light of the fact that one might well chose an ethic that is disapproved of by the community or the state. Africana religious figures in China who challenge the state's position on religious ideology are often apprehended and deported (Haugen, 2012). Even where the orientation is toward a neoliberal ethic, this proves also to be a source of ambivalence given that acquisitive tendencies tend to trump moral strictures (Crouch, 2016; Sen, 1989). Since communities, no matter how illiberal they are, have spaces for ethical resistance, the individual is ambivalent given the appeals to primordiality alongside the need for altruism, recognition, and restraint.

The modern individual—especially when of Africana heritage—is also wary of any community demands that under the guise of being ethical are in fact unethically limiting the possibilities for self-development. Especially vulnerable to such institutionalized disingenuousness are those with low skill levels who are embedded in weak and low-resource networks with transient lifestyles. They enact "cruel optimism," which Berlant's (2011) defines as modest acts of private generosity in neoliberal precincts that mask the reality of immobility and nurture the illusion of eventual upliftment. Low-skilled Africana workers in China in such a position lack the resources to be substantially interdependent in ways that are truly growth enhancing. To the degree that they are mobile, it is in the service of exiting from a bleak locale, to a similar bleak locale (Haugen, 2015). So while there is a caring ethos (Berlant, 2011) for these the most vulnerable, they lack the resource base and group support necessary to significantly improve their lot or to bring about systemic change.

Many Africana persons in China are embedded in transient communities with diverse subgroupings and varying commitments to each other, an arrangement that does not necessarily strengthen the ethical demands on the individual. As a result, self-development efforts are always at risk for being mediated by the individual's market-mediated narcissism rather than by a bracing ethical demand. Ambivalence again becomes the default position given the need for group support alongside the wariness of such support. Interestingly, despite the role that narcissism plays in such ambivalence, it also offers possibilities for ethical growth. This suggests that adaptive ambivalence guides the individual's commitment to figuring out how best to invest resources with regard to attempts for growth, recognition, reciprocation, and stability.

Given the diversity within the group, there is always the possibility of finding common cause with members committed to establishing safe places supportive of validating ethically informed efforts at self-growth and assisting others. One senses that such spaces exist within some of the unofficial ethnic churches and also in the social organizations that are part of the larger Africana communities. There is always uncertainty with its risk of failure and underachievement, but also, with group support, there is the possibility of making progress and having some gratifying sense of well-being. Such achievements are always difficult to achieve, anxiety is ever present, and ambivalence is a faithful shadow.

Traditional View of the Immigrant

Traditional academic perspectives of migrants portray them primarily as economic agents concerned with improving their material well-being (Haugen, 2012, 2015; Massey, 1990). Scant attention was paid to their subjectivities, and there was little disaggregation and recognition of their agency (Goss & Lindquist, 1995). In the post-World War II era, many immigrants did not leave out of fear of persecution but instead were economic migrants or sojourners (Conway, 2007; Selvon, 1989). Additionally, the focus was on south-to-north and east-to-west movements, with little attention to south-to-south flows.

Given that economic migrants often could not accumulate sufficient surplus to return to their respective home countries in a better financial position than when they had left, over time they mourned the loss of the original home and oriented toward the host country as their new home. For many of these migrants, including those of Africana heritage, ambivalence was present given, in part, the ambivalence directed at them by the host country. They were desired for their labor but often marginalized from the host communities due to their appearance and cultural differences; never experiencing a feeling of being fully accepted. For the political refugee, often fleeing to stay alive, ambivalence was also present, either as a function of being a negative *other* or from a reluctance to mourn the loss of the old and embrace the new (Said, 1993).

Theories on the emotional experience of migration have tended to focus on the experience as one of loss, finality, melancholy, and adaptation (Akhtar, 1995; Grinberg & Grinberg, 1982). The terms of separation with its murderous exclusion of those deemed *other* is dominant in psychoanalytic foundational thinking about migration and the *other*. It is embedded in a historical context of persecution and periodic expulsion, with little possibility of return.

Consequentially, psychoanalytic perspectives on migration are built on a foundation of the trauma of loss and the subsequent defensive coping responses. Grinberg and Grinberg (1982) formulate the issue as follows: "Migration as we have said comprises multiple traumas and involves numerous changes of external reality, with the subsequent repercussions on a person's inner reality" (p. 57). This is a reflection of studies of refugees by psychoanalysts who were themselves refugees, many of them fleeing the Holocaust, and the irretrievable loss of home and family. Such traumatizing flight makes nigh impossible the possibility of return (Shire, 2012). Given the finality of flight, immigrants are forced to reconfigure their internal world to be able to fully embrace a new home and identifications. This is a transitory phase, as integration comes about as the individual assimilates to the new home culture. Ambivalence therefore declines over time as a consequence of the decline in attachment to the original home (Akhtar, 1995).

From an intrapsychic perspective, immigrants must struggle with two sets of emotional identifications: one to the pre-immigration self and attachments, and another to the current self and its attachments to the host country. Assuming a substantive and positive attachment to the home country and also growing positive attachments to the new host country, immigrants are conflicted as they are experiencing both loss and exhilaration (Akhtar, 1995). The tendency might then be to engage in splitting; to denigrate the lost home as the price of privileging the host country. This is at best an initial short-term defense that can be adaptive, but if maintained over time, it acts as an impediment to the integrative work that the individual must do to resolve the conflict and to lower the degree of experienced anxiety (Walsh & Shulman, 2007).

Akhtar's (1995) presentation of an intrapsychic model of migration posits a third individuation. Based on Mahler, Pine, and Bergman's (2000) theory of separation-individuation, the child first individuates through the process of birth that causes physical separation from the mother. In the second individuation, children become aware that they are psychologically separate from the mother. Akhtar (1995) argues for an additional developmental step in which immigration is disruptive to preexisting relationships and ways of thinking of the self, given that the immigrant is not in the "average expectable environment" (p. 1052). In this place and through new relationships and self-perceptions, the immigrant develops what Akhtar refers to as, "New channels of self-expression become available. There are new identifications, different superego dictates, and different ideals" (p. 1052).

A psychoanalytic perspective is useful in certain ways despite its, at times, archaic and monochromatic approach to the subjectivities involved in migration. Psychoanalysis sensitizes us to the timelessness and animating urgency of desire, ever present, at best managed, never extinguished, and very much driving human endeavor including migration. It also offers a useful focus on the impact of prior experience on current ways of thinking and feeling, which in turn influences future actions. Immigrants, all too human, come with histories that have influence, often outside of awareness, on how they sculpt their futures. Contemporary theorists such as Mitchell (1993) speak to the multiplicity of components that constitute the self, often operating outside of consciousness, sensitivity to context, and the varied tactical approaches that inform their deployment:

> Yet selves change and are transformed continually over time; no version of self is fully present at any instant, and a single life is composed of many selves. An experience of self takes place necessarily in a moment of time; it fills one's psychic space, and other alternative versions of self, fade into the background.
>
> (p. 102)

The interplay between the economic and the affective is underprivileged in the standard literature, as much of migration research is focused on the migrants' need to acquire basic life-sustaining resources. Lacking is a well-differentiated sense of the immigrant with regard to curiosity, tenacity, and the ability to adapt to uncertainty. Frosh (2013) speaks to this lack: "There is no single identity, it is always open to the other, and claims for its univocality depend on drowning out the voices of the others that have given it shape" (p. 146).

In addition, neither the pleasures of leaving nor the possibility of return are really explored. Some immigrants had resources that allowed for reflection, agency, mobility, and the distinct possibility and intention of returning. Some spoke to the pleasures of exile, as it afforded them a place to enhance agency to reflect on traditional and limiting epistemologies that were then reconfigured in the service of self-improvement (Lamming, 1984; Said, 1993), while others appeared comfortable with their in-between-ness and were, in Said's (1993) evocative phrase, "happy with the idea of unhappiness" (p. 117). Beltsiou (2016) melds both Mitchell and Said when she notes: "Maybe coming home is befriending the fact that belonging is neither total nor constant, as we learn to inhabit our in-between spaces and come to settle between places" (p. 107).

A modern notion of progress, with its devaluation of the past and its emphasis on the future, left little space for the psychological oscillation, costs, and advantages represented by being in a state of in-between-ness. As such, there was not much sense of continuity between past and present. Schafer (2005), however, makes the point that in thinking about the individual's subjectivities, one starts not at the beginning but instead enters at the middle, that individuals are a part of something that has a history and a process that predates them, even as others also bring their history and process to that place. Schafer, although speaking in the context of a therapeutic relationship, makes the following observation that throws light on the experience of the migrant:

> They are already positioned in a host of contexts and prepared with volumes of anticipations, so that as much as they extend the borders of these contexts back in time and ahead into thinkable futures, and however they try to make them more inclusive, they never get free of their initial situatedness.
>
> (pp. 275–276)

So, Africana persons in China bring as part of their psyche, a history of both being constrained and being curious, but they also bring openness to new ways of perceiving, being in, and contributing to the world.

Thus the Africana person might well have experienced ambivalence given his or her reluctance to accept the limitations of home. Such individuals are often also embedded in networks that are linked to worldwide diaspora communities that both acknowledge ambivalence and have evolved strategies for effectively managing it. For some immigrants and foreign workers, ambivalence is fueled by the fact that all that is familiar is not necessarily overly chafing or substantively detrimental to growth, hence the adaptive ambivalence: not idealizing and yet not abandoning. When they leave, and when they are in the host country, foreigners are selective over time with what they privilege and what they marginalize (Jose, 2012).

Progressive Psychodynamic Positions on Migration: Bounded Hope

The contemporary world of migration is constantly changing, and there are progressive psychodynamic ways of understanding the psychological processes of migration. A new ease of communication and relatively low financial costs for transportation make it possible for some migrants to live materially and psychologically successful lives, embracing new identifications without entirely renouncing some significant aspects of old ones. These foreigners hover in a state of adaptive ambivalence with complex and ever-shifting identifications that are strategically deployed or withheld as a function of the psychosocial demands of the settings in which they are embedded and the goals they are pursuing.

Hoffman (2016) speaks to the normative nature of migration in the contemporary world:

> Migration, dislocation and various forms of nomadism are becoming the norm rather than the exception. It sometimes seems that

> lives rooted in one place and in a sort of narrative continuity are becoming the interesting aberration. But the extreme mobility that characterizes our world relativizes even the most stable identities. Even if we stay in one place, we know how easy it is to leave. Even if we live in countries with long histories and tradition, we are inescapably aware of the world's multiplicity and in most case the heterogeneity of our cultures. We know we are not the only centers of legitimacy.
>
> (pp. 214–215)

Such migrants in today's world do not feel the need to definitively renounce their homelands and cultures, even as they recognize the shortcomings that resulted in their leaving. Rather than the traditional model of loss and renunciation, Gonzalez (2016) suggests thinking of the host country as a transitional space, in a Winnicottian sense, that allows for the discovery and reconfiguration of the self. Such a space offers the possibility of accommodating and facilitating some of the realization of the foreign worker's dreams of self-development, while constraining others. Cecilia, a 31-year-old Ugandan investment advisor in Shanghai, noted:

> I developed myself more than anywhere else. I made more money. I am much stronger as a Black person. I am on the Metro, and no one wants to sit next to you, in the past I would have gotten mad. You see Whites and Chinese getting service before you. Over time I can live with this. I also learned to speak up for myself. My self-control is better. I think more for myself.

Those who adapt well to an irreducible ambivalence are able to respond effectively to contingencies, uncertainty, and opportunities that make for the possibility of self-growth through thoughtful risk taking. To the degree that they can manage social fluidity or, in Bauman's (2001) terms, liquid, multiple, and at times contradictory ways of engaging and being engaged, then there are possibilities for a sense of subjective well-being. In such an unstable world, with hierarchies in flux, the foreign worker is confronted with ontological questions and their attendant anxiety but also considerable amounts of opportunity.

As a consequence, the need to be attached has a noticeable contingent quality. These individuals have moorings, but these can be psychologically very utilitarian (Conway, 2007), with commitments undergoing frequent reassessment. Such an approach can, however, be emotionally costly, with many Africana persons in China bemoaning the lack of substantive relationships and the attendant loneliness given the peripatetic lifestyles they and their peers maintain.

Contemporary theories have begun to address some of these issues. Drawing on psychoanalytic theory, Akhtar (1995) proposes that loss of access to the relationships and concrete objects of the home country that have been intrinsic to subjectivity challenges the newcomer's psychic organization, creating a sense of flux reminiscent of earlier separation-individuation phases. As such, migration may trigger feelings pertaining to far earlier losses. At the same time, echoing Bhabha's (1994) notion of a "third space," Akhtar also argues that disruption can lead to psychic growth, to a "third individuation," as discussed a few pages ago. Altschuler (2008) notes that " it brings aspects of identity together in a different way, allowing for the development of an altered relationship with self, family and/or the nation" (p. 31).

Altschuler goes on to argue that there is always some sense of loss and pain that accompanies migration, and how that is managed can either obscure the psychological gains of migrating or can be so managed as to allow for new ways of configuring the self and relationships.

There is still an underlying assumption that the subject is an immigrant who has been accepted on a legally permanent basis into the new culture, alongside having a simultaneous loss of substantive access to the home culture. For many foreign individuals in host countries, including Africana workers in China, these are questionable assumptions. Many maintain daily contact through electronic media with emotionally significant others in the home country. In China, they face near insurmountable obstacles to becoming permanent residents and to being assimilated into Chinese communities. In such cases, ambivalence thrives, as while the contact with home can be emotionally enriching, individuals are also reminded as to why they chose to leave. Similarly, in China, they are constantly reminded of their otherness, but also of opportunities. These conditions do not facilitate the resolution of the substantive ambivalence that the individual experiences. At best, the individual is able to create adaptive approaches to its management.

Grinberg and Grinberg (1982) speak to this ambivalence when they note that the immigrant is dissatisfied with home but also is not comfortable in the host country given its intermittent hostility. They argue that being embedded in adequate networks and perceiving the self as competent and successful could assuage some aspects of this ambivalence. Assuming the presence of such qualities, then, an adaptive management of ambivalence can result in genuine self-growth. Akhtar (1995) notes that a mark of this achievement is the capacity and tendency of the individual to associate simultaneously and comfortably with individuals from both countries: "Such an identity, though perhaps lacking a deep anchoring in either historical-identification system, might yet possess a greater than usual breath of experience, a sense of relativity, knowledge, and at times, wisdom" (p. 1060).

No matter how adaptive, an ambivalent stance is costly for Africana persons in China, as it is extremely difficult to commit to a culture that is reluctant to accept immigrants. The foreigner cannot resolve the ambivalence but is left hovering between two worlds, attracted and skeptical toward both. At the same time, the foreigner must establish a sense of home, however transient; there must be some accommodation to belonging needs.

Adaptive Ambivalence: Recap

In China, as increasingly in other countries, the base response to some classes of foreign workers seems to be one of ambivalence. On the one hand, there is a desire for what that individual brings: labor, skills, and capital; on the other hand, there is wariness and sometimes hostility driven by concerns about their values and behaviors, as well as the demands they may place on the host culture. Some of these foreign workers assert themselves in terms of rights demands especially around recognition, social change, and support services. With such a reception, the immigrant might find it adaptive to maintain an ambivalent stance, given both attraction to and wariness toward the host country. Such a stance is almost inevitable in China given the practical impossibility of Africana persons, among other foreigners being granted permanent resident status. Well managed, this ambivalence permits self-growth that was not possible in the home country.

References

Adams, C. J. (2007). Respect and reputation: The construction of masculinity in poor African American men. *Journal of African American Studies*, *11*(3–4), 157–172.

Adams, C. J. (2015). Structure and agency: Africana immigrants in China. *Journal of Pan African Studies*, *7*(10), 85–108.

Akhtar, S. (1995). A third individuation: Immigration, identity and the psychoanalytic process. *Journal of the American Psychoanalytic Association*, *43*(4), 1051–1084.

Altschuler, J. (2008). Re-remembering and re-imagining relational boundaries: Sibling narratives and migration. *Annual Review of Critical Psychology*, *6*, 26–44.

Bauman, Z. (1991). *Modernity and ambivalence*. London, UK: Polity Press.

Bauman, Z. (2001). Identity in the globalizing world. *Social Anthropology*, *9*(2), 121–129.

Beltsiou, J. (2016). Seeking home in the foreign: Otherness and immigration. In J. Beltsiou (Ed.), *Immigration in psychoanalysis* (pp. 89–108). New York, NY: Routledge.

Berlant, L. (2011). *Cruel optimism*. Durham, NC: Duke University Press.

Bhabha, H. (1994). *The location of culture*. London, UK: Routledge.

Blumenthal, D., & Hsiao, W. (2005). Privatization and its discontents: The evolving Chinese health care system. *New England Journal of Medicine*, *353*, 1165–1170.

Conway, D. (2007). Caribbean transnational migration behavior: Reconceptualizing its "strategic flexibility." *Population, Space and Place*, *13*, 415–431.

Crouch, C. (2016). *The knowledge corrupters: Hidden consequences of the financial takeover of public life*. Cambridge, UK: Polity Press.

Fanon, F. (1967). *Black skin, white masks*. New York, NY: Grove Press.

Foster, R. (2016). The catastrophe of neo-liberalism: Finance, emancipation and disintegration. *Philosophy and Social Criticism*, *43*(2), 123–143.

Freire, P. (2000). *Pedagogy of the oppressed*. New York, NY: Continuum.

Freud, S. (1961). *Civilization and its discontents*. London, UK: W. W. Norton & Co.

Fromm, E. (1976). *To have or to be?* London, UK: Bloomsbury Academic.

Frosh, S. (2013). Psychoanalysis, colonialism, racism. *Journal of Theoretical and Philosophical Psychology*, *33*(3), 141–154.

Gonzalez, F. (2016). Only what is human can truly be foreign: The trope of immigration as a creative force in psychoanalysis. In J. Beltsiou (Ed.), *Immigration in psychoanalysis* (pp. 15–38). New York, NY: Routledge.

Goss, J., & Lindquist, B. (1995). Conceptualizing international labor migration: A structuration perspective. *International Migration Review*, *29*(2), 317–351.

Grinberg, L., & Grinberg, R. (1982). *Psychoanalytic perspectives on migration and exile*. New Haven, CT: Yale University Press.

Hairong, Y. (2003). Neoliberal governmentality and neohumanism: Organizing suzhi/value flow through labor recruitment networks. *Cultural Anthropology*, *18*(4), 493–523.

Hampson, N. (1990). *The enlightenment: An evaluation of its assumptions, attitudes and values*. London, UK: Penguin Books.

Haugen, H. (2012). Nigerians in China: A second state of immobility. *International Migration*, *50*(2), 65–80.

Haugen, H. (2015). Destination China: The country adjusts to its new migration reality. Retrieved from http://migrationpolicy.org/article/destination-china-country-adjusts-its-new-migration-reality

Hermans, H., & Dimaggio, G. (2007). Self, identity, and globalization in times of uncertainty: A dialogical analysis. *Review of General Psychology*, *11*(1), 31–61.

Hoffman, E. (2016). Out of exile: Some thoughts on exile as a dynamic condition. In Julia Beltsiou (Ed.), *Immigration in psychoanalysis* (pp. 211–215). New York: Routledge.

Joas, H. (2013). *The sacredness of the person: A new genealogy of human rights*. Washington, DC: Georgetown University Press.

Jose, E. (2012). The business plan. In A. Gardner & A. Watts (Eds.), *Constructing Qatar: Migrant narratives from the margins of the global system* (pp. 8–11). Retrieved from https://soundideas.pugetsound.edu/cgi/viewcontent.cgi?referer=www.google.com/&httpsredir=1&article=1735&context=faculty_pubs

Kashiwazaki, C., & Akaha, A. (2006). Japanese immigration policy: Responding to conflicting pressures. *Migration Policy Institute*. Retrieved from www.migrationpolicy.org/article/japanese-immigration-policy-responding-conflicting-pressures

Khanna, R. (2003). *Dark continents: Psychoanalysis and colonialism*. Durham, NC: Duke University Press.

Kleinman, A., Yan, Y., Jun, J., Lee, S., Zhang, E., Tianshu, P., ... Jinhau, G. (Eds.). (2011). *Deep China: The moral life of the person: What anthropology and psychiatry tell us about China today*. Berkeley, CA: University of California Press.

Lamming, G. (1984). *The pleasures of exile*. London, UK: Allison & Busby.

Levinas, E. (1985). *Ethics and infinity* (R. A. Cohen, Trans.). Pittsburgh, PA: Duquesne University Press.

Mahler, M., Pine, F., & Bergman, A. (2000). *The psychological birth of the human infant*. New York, NY: Basic Books.

Massey, D. (1990). The social and economic origins of immigration. *The Annals of the American Academy of Political and Social Science*, *510*, 60–72.

McGowan, T. (2016). *Capitalism and desire*. New York, NY: Columbia University Press.

Mitchell, S. (1993). *Hope and dread in psychoanalysis*. New York, NY: Basic Books.

Oishi, N. (2012). The limits of immigration policies: The challenges of highly skilled migration in Japan. *American Behavioral Scientist*, *20*(10), 1–21.

Russell, F. (1990). "Only something good can be evil": The genesis of Augustine's secular ambivalence. *Theological Studies*, *51*, 698–716.

Said, E. (1993). Intellectual exile: Expatriates and marginals. *Grand Street*, *47*, 112–124.

Schafer, R. (2005). Listening in psychoanalysis. *Narrative*, *13*, 271–280.

Selvon, S. (1989). *The lonely Londoners*. London, UK: Longmans.

Sen, A. (1989). Development as capability expansion. *Journal of Development Planning*, *19*, 41–58.

Senior, O. (2014). *Dying to better themselves: West Indians and the building of the Panama Canal*. Kingston, Jamaica: University of The West Indies Press.

Shire, W. (2012). Home. Retrieved from www1.villanova.edu/content/dam/villanova/mission/mandm... /Home.pdf

Smart, B. (1999). *Facing modernity: Ambivalence, reflexivity and morality*. London, UK: Sage Publications.

Strenger, C. (2016). *Freud's legacy in the global era*. New York, NY: Routledge.

Walsh, S., & Shulman, S. (2007). Splits in the self following migration: An adaptive defense or pathological reaction? *Psychoanalytic Psychology*, *24*(2), 355–372.

Wilkerson, I. (2010). *The warmth of other suns*. New York, NY: Vintage Books.

Wong, J. (2015, December 7). Beijing issues red alert over air pollution for the first time. *New York Times*. Retrieved from www.nytimes.com/2015/12/08/world/asia/beijing-pollution-red-alert.html

Zang, X. (2015). *Ethnicity in China: A critical introduction*. Malden, MA: Polity Press.

4 Modernity and Migration

Individuals are predisposed to inquire and to question and, given interdependencies, are embedded in groups that, if morally grounded, will attempt to tutor their imagination in a manner that is both gratifying and frustrating (Pruyser, 1983). The currently dominant capitalist ideology as well as the process of globalization facilitates a multiplicity of ways of being in the world, profoundly influencing the framework for the pursuit of recognition, as well as the development of cognitive and socio-emotional skill sets. This happens in the context of uncertainty given the absence of definitive ideologies (Bauman, 2001).

Modernity and its offshoot postmodernity create the ideological framework that is the midwife of capitalism, neoliberalism, and globalization. Its driving force is an insatiable curiosity fueled in part by logic and rationality in search of certainty. This logic fuels the insatiability of modernity, given its tendency to critique any given outcome, thereby driving further curiosity. It speaks to postmodernity, which can be thought of as modernity's skepticism toward its own transient certainties. Such relentless questioning give sensitizes individuals to differences generated by contingencies. They in turn fuel psychological states such as excitement, skepticism, anxiety, and ambivalence (Bauman, 1991).

Bauman (1991, 2001, 2003) portrays curiosity and modernity, as follows:

> Modernity is what it is—an obsessive march forward—not because it always wants more, but because it never gets enough; not because it grows more ambitious and adventurous, but because its adventures are bitter and its ambition is frustrated. The march must go on because any place of arrival is but a temporary station. No place is privileged, no place better than another, as from no place the horizon is nearer than from any other.
>
> (1991, p. 10)

Bauman is speaking to the insatiable quality of modernity, which has its genesis in human curiosity, which inevitably, generates means, such as technology, to ask even more discerning questions.

Features of Modernity

Curiosity

Human beings, unlike most other living creatures, are born with few sophisticated life-preserving skills. Their preeminent predisposition is the speed with which they can adapt to any given environment. Such a trait is crucial given the paucity of other predisposed survival skills, therefore requiring them to be thoughtful and vigilant. This vigilance is enhanced by curiosity being gratifying in and of itself. It enables the human subject to derive pleasure from explorations that are not tightly yoked to immediate needs gratification or survival. This is evident in some forms of migration that are not driven by fear, but by a desire to improve the self, and also a curiosity to explore the unknown. Such voluntary movements, especially of Africana persons, were evident in the post-World War II period, with many migrating to take advantage of economic and intellectual opportunities in Europe and North America, and relatively recently, of Africana persons into China.

This drive for improvement and less costly adaptation to a given place happened alongside the beginning of a sustained debate on human rights and human agency that resulted in the eventual demise of colonialism and the gradual retreat of archaic patriarchy. These changes generated a vast array of opportunities for individuals to explore, enabling them to reimagine themselves, and exercise agency in innovative and expansive ways.

Again, this curiosity emanates from the individual and over time becomes a contingency that if not independent of the individual is a major influence on self-definition. By way of illustration, persons of apparent Africana heritage have been recorded as visiting China over 1,500 years ago (Wyatt, 2009), and there is documentation of extensive contact between China and East Africa during the fifteenth century (Snow, 1988). Researchers such as Adams (2014, 2015); Bodomo (2012); Castillo (2015); Haugen (2012, 2015); Haugen and Diederich (2016a, 2016b, 2016c, 2016d, 2016e, 2016f); and Matthews (2011) have documented the initiatives, strategies, successes, and frustrations of Africana persons in China. Today, there are Africana traders and teachers of English in many areas of China, often the first of their kind seen in those precincts of relative ethnic homogeneity. They go for a variety of motives, with work, capital accumulation, and curiosity being the predominant ones. Some traders have steadily moved upmarket, eliminating the middle man, and in some cases buying their supplier.

This speaks to not just being satisfied with the status quo but observing, questioning, and initiating change, while also living with uncertainty.

Skepticism

The reflective component of modernity questions all posited certainties by emphasizing the inherently destabilizing role of contingency and the uncertainty, risk, and opportunity that it generates. The paradox is that even as modernity seeks certainty, in its postmodern presentation, it is skeptical of any perspective that makes claims to certainty. This, in turn, generates ambivalence given that opportunity is always accompanied by a degree of risk that can at best be managed, but never eliminated (Bauman, 1991). Through its constant questioning and its skepticism toward the grand and the holistic, modernism drives fragmentation, fuels doubts, and is the midwife of the tentative and the contingent. Such questioning creates spaces within which to exercise agency, be creative while building community, albeit at great struggle.

Bauman (1991) argues that while the assertion of agency makes the world seemingly manageable, it works against any grand vision where such visioning has historically resulted in curbs on the quality of imagination and the disciplining of the individual's dream. Modernity through its process of disaggregation of a given problem generates solutions that are locally acceptable, but it invariably generates new problems. A risk however is that the fragmentation of problem solving can result in a focus on the trivial instead of the profound, given the difficulty in conceptualizing a sustainable approach to the latter (Freire, 2000). Such fragmentation is a consequence of modernity's relentless, logic-based inquiry that has severely weakened long-standing ideological frameworks that informed and often constrained curiosity, self-gratification, and self-disciplining. Modernity's emancipation of individual agency is one of the main engines of migration that has resulted in thousands of Africana workers embedding themselves, however tentatively in China.

These processes of modernity offer both risk and opportunity, so the individual socialized into certainty and who is averse to risk taking and its attendant anxiety may have difficulty fully seizing a given opportunity. Such an individual may instead be immobilized by focusing on risk and the absence of certainty and clear guidelines. The difficult but necessary quest for an organizing vision embedded in a supportive structure therefore sits alongside dissatisfaction with what is often experienced. This can be tolerated and even relished as a challenge for the resilient and well-supported individual.

Such unfettering came at a cost, as the lack of certainty generated high levels of anxiety given the drastic decline of definitive ideologies. This includes the risk of spiritual emptiness, amorality, and the consumption of drugs, material goods, and sex in futile attempts at assuaging the anxiety that uncertainty engenders. For many, questions of recognition and belonging came into sharp relief, and even as they exercised new-found agency, it was difficult to get definitive answers.

Risk management is evident among some Africana persons in China who minimize risk taking by limiting their interactions to other non-Chinese expatriates or Chinese persons with a Western orientation. Others may appear to embed in Chinese communities but remain on the periphery given their reluctance to master the Chinese language. For both groups, curiosity about China and the possibilities for self-development are only modestly engaged. Others will leap before they look, often with good outcomes given a broad suite of capabilities including high levels of resilience and the requisite social, intellectual, and technical skill sets.

Agency and Contingency

The search for certainty is thought to be in the service of improving life chances. While the literature on migration has stressed economic opportunities, theorists such as de Haas (2014) have sensitized us as to the role that aspirations beyond the material animate the behavior of migrants. An increasingly globalized ease of movement and access to knowledge allows for the questioning of dominant and historically oppressive epistemologies. These consequences of modernity have created space for more autonomous individuality that in turn facilitates an increased awareness of subjectivity and its creative expression. The resultant weakening of the hold of the group over the individual allows for greater attempts at self-improvement and increased mobility. So in China, the millions of Chinese people moving to the cities of the east coast to satisfy the need for labor are responding to similar psychological aspirations and market forces as many of the Africana workers in China (Castillo, 2015). However, such increased autonomy can also lead to a sense of alienation, as well as the attenuating of the ethical constraints that apply to individuals with the attendant risk of unhealthy levels of narcissism. These changes endanger the possibility of sustenance that comes from a healthy community and loosens the constraints on capitalist predations.

Being more knowledgeable and rational equips the individual with the skill sets necessary to negotiate a world of opportunity and risk that lacks a central organizing ethos. The same world that is a place of opportunity and risk is also a world in which impersonal market forces are dominant inasmuch as they comprise an orienting, albeit amoral, ethos, given the retreat of the state as a regulatory, nurturing, and protective actor (Bauman, 1991). Such an ethos, while generating a wide range of opportunities, at the same time creates systems that make for uneven access to the resources necessary to take advantage of those opportunities (Crouch,

2016). For countless decades, exposed in their home countries or minority communities to possibilities alongside the lack of resources to exploit those opportunities, many Africana persons, among others, have left home in search of more resource-friendly spaces (Senior, 2014; Wilkerson, 2010).

From a historical and contemporary perspective, for many Africana persons, modernity and the rampant capitalism and accelerated globalization that are its offspring have been a mixed blessing, bringing much uncertainty and loss of community and little in the way of enhanced agency and wealth. Modernity, with its intellectual and technology facilitated products, has unleashed skepticism and moral ambiguity that unwittingly facilitated the industrialization of the Atlantic slave trade, and it also facilitated the colonization of huge swathes of the Africana world and its exploitation and underdevelopment (Rodney, 2011; Williams, 1994). This of course introduced uncertainty without the opportunities.

Ethical Decoupling

Africana persons in China find themselves having both left a home country struggling to find its ideological true north and embedding in a China in the throes of a similar struggle. Some come with adaptive skills honed from being peripatetic foreign workers, and they also bring deep anxieties about the meaning of home and about ways of measuring growth that are not limited to the cognitive, technical, and the material. All struggle with the ethics of relating to other Africana persons and to Chinese peers.

According to Bauman (1991), a challenge of modernity is congruent with Joas' (2013) position that central to any ethical approach is the perspectives of the individual. This is in contrast to the more traditional position that limits the individual to simply aligning their views to that of the status quo and its illusion of certainty. Inherent in modernity are flux and mobility that constantly question all constraints whether they are scientific, artistic, or moral. Inherent in the curiosity that drives the modern is also the questioning of that which it encounters, thereby changing the observed and then moving on. Such a posture destabilizes the certainty that modernity seeks to find and by extension questions all ethical positions. This decoupling is a consequence of a circular process, whereby reflective individuals interrogate their epistemological frameworks that in turn grant them greater deference and agency, that in turn make them question more. Such an approach does not validate and therefore creates a moral vacuum that is often filled by a disingenuously crafted ethic in the service of self-interest constrained at best by fear of sanctions against commitment to an increasingly elusive well-grounded morality. It also speaks to the ever-present conflict that humans experience in the wish to be nurtured and protected, with its necessary constraints, and the wish to be unfettered and impulsive.

The Africana person in China must be quite vigilant on ethical matters given the risk of being exploited or being tempted to engage in unethical practices. These can occur within his Africana networks or in his interactions with various Chinese individuals and institutions. It can also originate in his family where members may place unreasonable demands or might not reciprocate in ways asked of them.

Given the opportunities and risk that this highly contingent mix of structure and agency generates, many persons cross borders to flee oppression or to realize a dream. For Africana foreign workers in China, among others, as we have seen, ambivalence is a permanent psychological condition, a consequence of the ever-present tension between the benefits and costs of their attempts to improve themselves. The successful individual learns to adapt to exercise agency within constraints and to manage the anxieties inherent in living in an at times fluid and at other times rigid social milieu. The relentless inquiry of modernity, the rapaciousness and creativity of capitalism, and the myriad effects of globalization are challenging to individuals. These forces interacting with individuals' predispositions, and the quality of their group support profoundly shape how Africana persons in China, among others, engage in self-making.

Overview of Migration

People have been migrating for eons, starting with ancient ancestors who migrated out of Africa. It is estimated that 3.2 percent of the world's current population or over 200 million persons engage in some form of migration (United Nations Department of Economic and Social Affairs Population Division, 2013). Such movements reflect the subjectivities of the individual such as curiosity, the quest for self-improvement, or the flight from danger. They also reflect the impact of structural processes such as increasingly globalized and affordable access to technologies of communication and travel, declining birth rates in the developed countries, and the increasing demand for transnational labor and talent.

The migration process inevitably generates conflictual relationships at the individual and group level that reflect the ambivalence of the various actors. So, the lack of opportunity at home alongside the lack of substantive recognition can engender feelings of frustration, alongside deeply felt regret in some at having to migrate. In the host country, the conflict that speaks to the ambivalence is often the demand for foreign labor, alongside a hostile visa regime and an ambivalent community reception. These ambivalent interactions contribute to a self-making and migration process that is psycho-socially demanding. From a socioeconomic perspective, there is a fluidity and diversity to the way individuals move around in a globalized world and how they are recognized in various host countries.

Vignette: Mikhaila

About Mikhaila

Mikhaila is a 29-year-old of Jamaican and American heritage whose tertiary education took place in Jamaica (undergraduate), the United States (MBA), and China (further post-graduate studies); she has been living in China for the past 4 years. She is based in Shanghai, where she works both as a corporate trainer and also as an entrepreneur who owns a personal services company in Shanghai that caters to Africana clients. She decided to come to China following the beginning of the 2008 recession in the United States, where there was little work to be had. To do this, she did research online and then located work in Shanghai and a West Indian network there that helped her to adjust. Mikhaila is neither fluent nor literate in Chinese.

Mikhaila likes her lifestyle in China, perceiving it as a place of limitless opportunity, even it can be exasperating:

> It is like a rollercoaster here. At one moment you are excited at an accomplishment, and the next moment you are questioning why you are staying here. You are denigrated because of the color of your skin as when people will not shake your hand. Then men will approach you on the street and compliment you. Your days are full of surprises.

Mikhaila has had to struggle with racist and sexist behavior in China, manifested as being passed over for consulting assignments in favor of White men from the West:

> I think it is less racist here than what I experienced in Manhattan (New York). The Chinese are very friendly even if they are often racist. Racism is not overt in China. The culture of "face" means they cannot show they are racist as they will lose face, so racism is not shown directly. They do it in small ways. If you go to buy shoes they will tell you they "do not carry Black people shoes," meaning large sizes. Another example is when you send in a glowing resume with your picture because they need to know you are not Black. You must be White with blue eyes.

She also noted a hierarchy of race with Whites first and Africans at the bottom. Yet she thinks racism is less embedded in the Chinese compared to the United States, where she found racism more pervasive and enduring. She found that in her interactions with many Chinese people, they were willing to change their perceptions once they got to know her, noting that the perception of a Black person as smart or talented such as Obama and Usain Bolt would trump a previous negative view of Blackness.

Mikhaila is both challenged and troubled by the tenor of business relationships in China:

> They are not to be trusted as they are very patriotic and insular. If you are an outsider, they privilege China; they will use you. If you are getting ahead here, its only because it is benefiting them. They like cunningness in others, and they will therefore admire you if you bargain hard.

She is excited by China's competitive atmosphere but struggles to come to terms with the prevalence of dishonesty and corruption. She argues that being both Africana and female requires a degree of vigilance and intellectual acuity given the tendency of many Chinese businesspersons to perceive her as inferior. As a corporate trainer, she works with Chinese managers who are well schooled in Western business practices yet in subtle ways are always oriented toward Chinese interests and ways of doing business.

Mikhaila feels she has matured considerably since coming to China:

> I am no longer carefree. I am better at dealing with things myself; at making emotional and financial decisions. I am answerable to myself. I used to call my mother a lot with problems. Now I deal with them myself; I am on my own.

She does not envisage a long-term stay in China, given the visa challenges, the limitations of the religious community, and the difficulty in finding a partner.

Mikhaila's lifestyle embodies the opportunities and risks of an Africana person in China during this period of globalized capitalism in late modernity. Mikhaila is embedded in multiple and resource-rich networks, in part as a result of her ethnic roots but also as a function of being skilled, credentialed, reflective, and discerning. As is often the case with successful foreign workers, she is a highly qualified and experienced transnational worker who is therefore able to deploy a range of skill sets acquired across a variety of different cultural and business settings. This has contributed to a resiliency that allows her to cope with difference when it presents as an obstacle and to embrace it when it offers the possibility of enriching her life.

The Immigrant Individual in the Contemporary World: The Ceaseless Quest of Modernity and the Rotating Lens of Postmodernity

Mikhaila feels a strong emotional attachment to Jamaica, her home country, and to a lesser extent to New York, where many family members have relocated:

> From the age of eight, I moved back and forth a lot between New York and Jamaica. So in some ways I have two homes. My heart is in Jamaica, but I am not sure I will ever be able to live there again. The lifestyle that I have gotten used to in China, I cannot have in Jamaica. It is safe here [in Shanghai]; my guard is lowered here. It is easy, there is no crime. That is important for a woman.

As a result, her ideas of home have changed:

> Home used to be where your family was. Now it is how you transition into somewhere where you are comfortable; it is in your comfort zone. As you mature, home is what you make it. It is not just about family, but also friendships.

This evolving view sits alongside a still keenly felt love of Jamaica and a commitment to help her home country and the Caribbean region in whatever way she can. Mikhaila aspires to facilitate the sale of Caribbean products in China.

Mikhaila has clear-eyed views of the challenges she faces and some of the conflicts that she must manage. Her ambivalence with regard to her home country reflects a conflict between emotionally positive experiences alongside awareness of its dangers and limitations. The compromise for her is to maintain a distance and relinquish thoughts of settling there. Home for her becomes a complex amalgamation of memories of experiences from different developmental periods with varying affective investments. It also speaks to contemporary needs for a psychologically stable base from which to launch and work on self-projects, and finally, it speaks to mature melancholy: experiences that can be treasured of a place and time that can never be recovered. Mikhaila finds, despite her conflict, that her love of her "original" home is as strong as ever and thinks of ways in which to express and nurture her affection through acts of assistance.

China provides an almost mirror opposite set of attractions and limits. It is a site for Mikhaila to develop her capacities as a businessperson and to learn to entertain a wider sense of difference. As such, she feels a sense of having grown in terms of her intellectual skills, her ability to tolerate, and at times the capacity to embrace difference. She struggles to negotiate an ever-shifting ethical landscape hampered by her lack of close relationships with Chinese nationals, and her limited Chinese language fluency. This has also hampered her ability to build enduring and ethically informed interdependent relationships with Chinese nationals outside the sphere of business.

While Mikhaila is comfortable exploring a diverse range of cultural settings, she struggles to find a perspective that will enable her to make sense of the at times contradictory responses she garners as an Africana woman in China. In classic postmodern style, she has a hodgepodge of ways of thinking about difference in China, accompanied by the ambivalence emanating from her inability to resolve the central dilemma of having no place where she feels fully recognized and at the same time is able to fully exercise her sense of agency.

Resistance to Capitalism's Grip as Expression of Agency

Mikhaila is very sociable and has friends across the non-Chinese racial and ethnic spectrum: "Africans and Europeans tend to stick with their own groups, but I transcend that type of relating. I move between all the groups, and that is unusual." She is in some ways the informal mayor of the Africana community in Shanghai as head of an Africana-oriented community organization that is inclusive of both Africana and Western individuals and their diverse sensibilities. The organization stages social events to facilitate networking and cultural solidarity. In addition, it offers tutoring and some welfare services to children and families of Chinese internal immigrants, a group that is often disparaged and marginalized in large urban centers such as Shanghai.

Mikhaila is embedded in a Chinese culture where market values are widely accepted but are in tension with cultural values such as tradition and nationalism and with human needs for intimacy, spirituality, and community. There is a strongly expressed wariness of the seemingly unfettered and narcissistic individual that is odd given the exhortations for individuals to be creative and show initiative. At the same time, the seemingly selective Chinese embrace of capitalism results in it being difficult to articulate a stable and acceptable epistemology that can nurture community, while promoting creativity, and the skepticism that comes with it. It is difficult in such a setting, with its history of authoritarianism in collision with a skeptical modernism, to find safe places to explore spirituality and intimacy without the intrusion of either the state or the market.

There are possibilities for resistance as an expression of the adaptive use of an ever-present sense of ambivalence. Mikhaila is committed to sustained acts of assistance in a diverse set of domains. In the case of her business, she has succeeded in creating and running a profitable business out of assisting peers and building community. Mikhaila is pragmatic about the possibilities and limits in China and will eventually leave. As she and so many other foreign workers have noted: China is not a final destination. She is more assured about herself than she was prior to coming to China. She is unclear as to where the future will take her but is confident that she has the skills, resilience, and support to continue to grow and to exercise her agency in ways that are rewarded and gratifying.

Advantages of Uncertainty

Some forms of uncertainty are not without its advantages. It can result in commitment to a process that is inspired by a vision that might well not be achieved but the pursuit of which can give meaning and a sense of continuity (Smart, 1999). This is evident with Mikhaila who celebrates the chances available in China but does not miss the uncertainty around personal safety in Jamaica.

One would need safeguards to ensure that the pursuit of self-development is neither an act of cruel optimism nor a task that requires the individual to be a superhuman being. When grounded in a reasonable code of ethics flowing from ethically informed individuals, it offers both reasonable autonomy and the acceptance of necessary constraints. Given the uncertainty, the vision for oneself needs constant renewal and ideally an ethically informed and resilient capacity to reflect.

Ambivalence

To be human is to be ambivalent about the necessity of interdependence and the attendant ethical demands and its inherent constraints. These are always viewed warily by the individual who both wishes to be unfettered and also to be nurtured and protected. As a consequence, one can sometimes observe a pattern of selective withdrawal into the self and a corresponding lack of concern for the public sphere (Smart, 1999). Group involvement and commitment, no matter how affectively intensive, is utilitarian given the ultimate focus is on the self. The individual is often reluctant to be in situations that require offering assistance to others in the absence of any benefit accruing to him or her (Bauman, 2003). Such a narcissistic stance is troubling as it limits the space for ethical behavior that is the basis of morality, given the lessening of personal interaction, of mutual recognition, and of interdependencies.

So, while individuals are freed from the stasis of certainty, they must cope with the ambivalence that manifests itself as the exhilaration with the seemingly infinite range of opportunities available in tension with the ever-present anxiety fueling the search for a stabilizing, albeit tenuous, ethos. There are therefore multiplicities of centers that arbitrate difference and privilege positions and, therefore, no definitive way of deciding which center to orient toward—assuming the individual has a choice.

Affective commitments and tradition can limit self-development. By way of contrast dispassion, as a function of dissatisfaction with tradition as limits on self, combined with ambivalence, could make the individual orient toward other centers of influence that facilitate self-development. Yet there is never a view from nowhere, as the individual is never without a cultural compass, despite some awareness of its inherently biased readings. Cultural spaces that deploy regulatory regimes that are morally informed and facilitate ethical interpersonal interactions are an important bulwark against the dehumanization and nihilism that might come with an unduly unbounded life.

For the Africana person in China, ambivalence is a lived experience that might be managed in adaptive if costly ways. Individuals such as Mikhaila exult in emerging themselves in a China that is intellectually and materially enriching, resulting in experiences that have made them more knowledgeable, discerning, and self-assured. At the same time, they must struggle with the realization that they might never be fully accepted in a Chinese community and that they carry their own antipathies to China, especially with regard to issues of ethics, community, and creativity.

Africana Possibilities

For Africana people in China, postmodernity's unceasing inquiry offers the possibility of deploying dispassion to understand their ontological legacy, especially in relation to their keenly felt consumption yearnings with regard to knowledge and material gain. Many Africana persons have histories of being embedded in structures that constrained agency across intellectual, political, and economic spheres. Such limits on self-development were somewhat assuaged by being in caring communities that tolerated the restlessness of the individual who questioned and sought more than knowledge and goods.

Coming to China offered the possibility of being relatively unfettered in the pursuit of technical knowledge and wealth. This access required the individual to accept the frustration arising from the uncertainty and constraints around developing a more holistic vision that could also encompass ethical interdependencies and the support of a diverse and moral community. China for such an individual exemplifies the features of late modernity as it offers opportunity and, in the face of uncertainty, re-feudalist and regressive risks.

In summary, modernity has conditionally freed the individual from the suffocating and self-limiting stasis of the premodern world. With its relentless questioning posture, it allows the modern individual to actualize and manage heretofore rich scenarios around self in the world. Such unfettering of the imagination and unrelenting questions are not without risks. These shifts have created spaces where being ethical appears to be optional and therefore individuals are at risk of being exploited and victimized. Such potential outcomes suggest that there is a hovering risk of a return to the limitations on self-development that many Africana workers thought would not be as prevalent in China.

Features of Capitalism

In its most basic sense, capitalism is an ideology that places an emphasis on the growth of capital resources as a worthy goal in and of itself. This is best done by engaging the self-interest of individuals by rewarding their willingness to take risks and be creative in the context of competing with other like-minded individuals. Such an approach, with its urgency and restlessness, facilitates skepticism toward stasis and is the engine of material prosperity. It is this possibility of enhancing agency and therefore improving their position in life that fuels the dreams of many of the persons who leave home on a quest for self-improvement.

Capitalism, however, has no inherent morality and can be considered a hired gun that, depending on how it is deployed, can enhance agency and community or severely constrain the first and weaken the second. This is evident in what Crouch (2016) terms *post-democracy*, a phase marked by the decline of individual agency, difficulty in building solidarity, and a sense that once democratic cultures are becoming pre-democratic. In such a state, the members of the ruling class become the capitalists, and, given their focus on capital accumulation, they offer shallow enchantment, hollow community, and autonomy geared toward consumption.

So, in its current dominant form, capitalism can be quite destructive, as it is often in the service of our most primitive, aggressive, and pleasure-seeking instincts. Slavery and human trafficking are perhaps the most egregious example of unbounded capitalism. Within the Africana community in southern China, one can observe examples of the pursuit of self-interest and profit among some of its members, as manifested in the many visa scams run by Africana persons in complicity with corrupt Chinese administrators. Africana businesspersons also report the need for vigilance with regard to quality when ordering goods for export from some Chinese manufacturers, given the unethical tendency to substitute low-quality ware for the high-quality ware that was ordered (Bodomo, 2012).

Upon exposure to a capitalist ideology that places emphasis on immediacy, seemingly unfettered agency, and consumption, the individual is at risk for deploying a form of agency that is unhealthy and ultimately limits agency. Here, however, the limits are in part a function of the absence of positive and socially based constraints that can protect the individual against the temptation to be defensively primitive by deploying agency. Capitalism often limits the capacity of the group to conceive and enforce positive social limits that can protect individuals against the self-damaging nature of their instincts in the context of a world of increasing complexity, ambiguity, and unpredictability (Hermans & Dimaggio, 2007). In China, with the temptations of materialism, the unevenness of ideological guidelines, selective negative constraints, and the tenuousness of community, the unthoughtful deployment of agency is a constant risk for the individual. This is in addition to the everyday reality of having to deal with individuals engaging in unethical behavior.

Individuals in the modern world can therefore find themselves in positions where their creative energies, under the influence of a capitalist ideology embedded in the social unconscious, are in the service of appealing to the primordial aspect of being human. So, for example, for many Africana persons in China, the attraction speaks to knowledge acquisition at times in tension with the thoughtless pursuit of material wealth. Without reflection and discipline, the individual is often yoked to a mindless and increasingly costly pursuit of pleasure through consumption. Given these links to our primitivity, capitalist ideologies are often deployed in opposition to time and consumption constraints, to group life, and to being reflective. Although many Africana persons are proud of their intellectual and material accomplishments in China, many bemoan the lack of community and the limits on spiritual development that are features of living under an illiberal regime that embraces selective aspects of a capitalist ideology.

Capitalism, Ideology, and Uncertainty

Capitalism is, however, quite protean, and when appropriately regulated, it is a force for motivation and facilitating being reflective, creative, and agentic. So, disciplined Africana persons in China are often able to generate and deploy their surplus to improve their quality of living and to facilitate a less financially precarious future. Where dominant and therefore relatively unfettered, however, capitalism often leaves little space for ideologies that address issues of the good life that are not reduced to material wealth and consumption (Binkley, 2011). A central paradox of capitalism is that it is an ideology that marginalizes other ideologies that are important in the quest for holistic living—a goal that capitalism purports to support. This tendency, by the vacuum it creates, engenders a sense of uncertainty and often anxiety in the average person This is the consequence of their being a paucity of models that speak to the construction of healthy subjectivities that are not reduced to an over-reliance on reasoning, the never-ending acquisition of technical skills, and a preoccupation with consumption. For Africana persons in China, there is often a sense of an uncomfortable pact that leaves them feeling that they must adapt to being always ambivalent given the sense of incompleteness whether at home, in China, or anywhere else in a world dominated by capitalism. While it can assuage certain needs, capitalism often unwittingly brings into sharp relief the need states it cannot address.

The individual's sense of incompleteness is exacerbated by an important and potentially debilitating effect of capitalist ideology on the psychology of agency. In its current iteration, it has reduced the role of the state from a body that nurtures and protects the individual to one that instead forces the individual to cede authority to market forces and the community of financiers. Many Africana persons come from cultures of weak governance, where market forces and rentiers dominate with a resultant marked economic and political inequality. The flight to China, while offering some maneuverability, also results them embedding in a space with its own market-based and ideological limits on personal agency. In such settings, there is little buffer against the uncertainty of the marketplace and the indifferent, if not hostile, state. For Africana persons in China who are not skilled and are not embedded in well-resourced support groups, uncertainty represents not opportunity but pain and a diminution of already modest amounts of agency (Haugen & Diederich, 2016a, 2016b, 2016c, 2016d, 2016e, 2016f).

Many Africana persons in China reveal a pattern of acquiring knowledge and some wealth and then being somewhat perplexed as to their next move, given ambivalence about either returning home or living in China. Those developed skill sets are the building blocks of a healthy self, but without attention to the spiritual and socio-emotional aspects of the self, the individual is left vulnerable to mimicking a heavily promoted style of living that leads to the creation of false aspects of the self.

Ontological anxiety is further caused by an abundance of cultural transmissions, given that within a range of options the individual lacks any definitive guidelines in self-construction. Categories such as gender, sexuality, and citizenship are open to an increasing range of interpretations that make self-construction an exercise in fluidity and uncertainty, with each interpretation having a counter interpretation and an absence of definitive positions given that such positions are themselves contested (Bauman, 2001). This contributes to ambivalence as individuals perceive both pleasure and dread in any given position they may adopt in the process of fashioning the self. In this regard the Chinese space is often a replica of the original home space with regard to attitudes to sexuality. Africana persons who are not heterosexual report caution in exploring their sexuality for fear of social disapproval and vulnerability to not having their visas renewed.

Globalization: Capitalism's Enigmatic Handmaiden

Globalization is the process of disseminating on a worldwide basis an ideology such as capitalism, and related ways of thinking such as market-based ideation, as the ideal arbiter of value and worth. Multimedia messages, remittances, and the lifestyles of returning Africana workers to their respective home countries are conduits for disseminating the virtues of a capitalist lifestyle.

Facilitated by mass media, globalization also privileges ways of self-construction such as particular types of cognition, for example, unhealthy consumption processes that emphasize taste, while marginalizing the importance of nutrition. Such thinking also privileges individual agency at the cost of group life. Capitalism's influence over mass media means that certain ways of constructing the self are presented as normative as opposed to being presented as only a few of a great many choices, and these limited ideas about self-construction thus go on to dominate and distort the globalization process. This process is often the principal means of disseminating practices that will maximize capital production and increase surplus, often to the detriment of healthy subjectivities and a sense of being safe.

Globalization as Counter-Hegemonic: The Paradox of Capitalism in Relationship to Globalization

Given that globalization is not an ideology but is a very efficient means of spreading ideologies, it is also the means by which counter-narratives to the capitalistic, Western-influenced models can be disseminated. Therefore inherent in globalization is a powerful paradox. Capitalism's appeal to the primordial can often increase the will to agency that in turn can energize reflective tendencies and a resistance to the capitalist temptation to enact a shallow and false self. Given the relative unregulated nature of the internet, messages that promote capitalism must compete with those that advocate a more thoughtful and less consumerist and narcissistic approach to living. The discerning individual might well find the tools to limit capitalist aggressions using the same globalized communication networks that seek to promote such actions. Some Africana persons in China, facilitated by social media networks, devote considerable time and other resources to assist both Chinese and Africana persons in need. Such actions, they report, re-animate their sense of themselves as being part of a nurturing community and widens their experience of both Chinese and fellow Africana persons.

Resistance to Disenchantment

Such cultural bricolage offers the possibility of a resistance to disenchantment and a resurgence of spirituality as evidenced by fairly high engagement in religious activities by Africana persons in China. This is engaged in at some risk, given the wariness of the Chinese authority to spiritual-based community organizations. The Africana person in China must manage in an adaptive way the ambivalence that globalization engenders through the offering of seemingly infinite and often conflicting choices. It offers opportunities as it makes possible meaning-making and creativity on a scale and depth hereto unimaginable. At the same time, it also offers much temptation to develop and enact false selves characterized by unthoughtful consumption of both goods and commodified and shallow ontologies. This can trigger complex and contradictory impacts on self-making and identity. These structural elements make for an ambivalent self, a deep-seated sense of ontological insecurity.

Historical Objectification and Commodification of the Africana Body

Of especial relevance is capitalism's significance as a dominant ideology that has profoundly shaped societies and self-construction on a worldwide basis for over 500 years. Specific to persons of Africana heritage is the objectification of Africana persons as bodies purely in the service of labor and illicit pleasure and their subsequent enslavement, with scant regard for their humanity and the attendant limits on their agency and voluntary mobility. This commodifying of Africana persons resulted in their surplus value being extracted and invested outside of the colonies or communities in which they resided. This deliberate under-investment in institutions for the development of Africana persons in Africa and its diaspora communities created economic circumstances that made migration to places with resources inevitable. The pursuit of self-development through migration is an unavoidable consequence of a rampant capitalism and is a defining characteristic of most Africana communities. A consistent theme in Africana persons' stories in China is the necessity of leaving home due to lack of educational opportunities and lack of meaningful and well-paying work.

Modernity, Migration, and the Self

Contemporary markets are increasingly a reflection of a globalized capitalism and the related opportunities and constraints that the individual must effectively manage. With economies in uneasy dependence on each other and a seemingly insatiable market for novelty and innovative processes, there is a worldwide hunt for individuals who are talented and skilled. While such individuals fuel capitalism, they also offer ethical alternatives to capitalist practices.

Such individuals are in short supply and command hefty premiums and attractive working conditions. China is in the market for such highly mobile workers, but given its antipathy to the outsider, it is ambivalent with regard to how much mobility it gives to them. It has recently promulgated immigration laws that allow for the granting of "creative" visas, available to individuals like the many Africana persons working in high status jobs that add value to goods and services produced. At the same time, Chinese officials have been making it more difficult for low-skilled foreign workers to stay in China.

Ideally, the individual whose capabilities are attractive to the market will experience high degrees of mobility; de Haas (2014) defines mobility in terms of the freedom to choose where to live and where to move to, combined with the capability to do so. Of special relevance to Africana persons in China, mobility, in de Haas' formulation, includes the freedom to stay. Of course, such freedom in China is constrained by the dominance of its temporary visa stance for the overwhelming amount of foreigners living there, regardless of their capabilities. Using Franquesa's (Van Hear, 2014) concept of mobility being on a continuum from mobile to immobile, Africana workers in China, regardless of income, value-added, status, or length of legal stay, struggle to manage where they fall over time on the immobility/mobility continuum. This speaks ultimately to the limitation on agency placed on foreign workers despite the capitalist-driven need for their services. In such an often ethically challenged marketplace, the individual must find or establish and nurture a community that can exploit the self-enriching possibilities of modernity, while at the same time provide a buffer against its capitalistic and anomie-inducing disingenuous offerings. Increasingly, individuals deploy their mobility to find hospitable places to adaptively manage this uncertainty-generating paradox. In Guangzhou, African workers invest much resource in developing and sustaining trustworthy business relationships. This is necessary given that there is no legal recourse if a contract is not honored. Similarly, in Shanghai peer support is necessary to decipher the nuanced ways of interacting and deploying creative skills in the typical Chinese corporate setting.

Many Africana workers in China are able to successfully work on keenly felt developmental needs alongside an awareness of other needs that have been marginalized. Many report that at some risk they attend illegal churches that address their need for substantive spiritual nurturance. There is often the realization that what is keenly desired might well be either very costly or unattainable. As we saw in Chapter 3, under such conditions of constraint and uncertainty, ambivalence is inevitable.

In such market and community settings, access to timely information as well as access to global Africana networks enriches the capacity of the individual to make informed choices in the service of self-development. Successful Africana persons in China are embedded in such networks that buffer them against dubious sources and practices while giving them access to authenticated information and ways of being. As noted earlier, these networks are biased toward cognitive and professional development and are less helpful with regard to emotional challenges.

Such access increases the possibility of the individual being more discerning in thinking and more tolerant in encounters with difference. This in turn contributes to increased possibilities of success at certain aspects of self-building (Adams, 2014; Martin & Sugarman, 2000). The exposure to such a wide range of information, in combination with the individual's subjectivity, allows for creative interpretations around self and ways of being more effective in the world. The contingencies generated offer the possibility of new ways of interpreting personal history and of understanding the self, its vulnerabilities, and its possibilities (Martin & Sugarman, 2000). Some Africana persons joyfully exploited the refreshing and at times startling reorientation of some aspects of their worldview. One woman noted that she had begun to develop an appreciation of how the world was understood from a non-Western perspective. Others commented on having a more nuanced and broader sense of Africa based on their exposure to Africana persons from the continent.

Consideration must be given to the often-unstated expectation that the Africana person will fulfill the dreams of those left behind and contain the traumas they experienced and yet not overly dissociate from the home culture and its constraints. Partly motivating those hopes are an adaptive distancing from and an overcoming of the constraining legacies of the home culture such as family, community, and historical constraints. The individual acknowledges those legacies but resists their essentialist-driven gravitational pull. The attraction of modernity with its disdain for history and its exhortation to embrace reinvention and self-development is both exciting and a source of anxiety and creates yet another challenge calling for managing ambivalence in an adaptive manner.

The Africana person in China, being in a context of multiple cultures, must deploy different aspects of the self in response to opportunity, narcissistic injuries, and the possible re-experiencing of race-based trauma. In dealing with these challenges, Bodnar (2004) evokes the possibility that the individual's prior history can be both help and hindrance. It is worth remembering that the roots of the Africana person's ambivalence lie in the home country with the character-marked history of gratification and frustration. That history also speaks to a degree and quality of reflective capacity resulting in a determination to leave that may or may not be well informed by an unblinking assessment of individual strengths and weaknesses. The psychological need to dis-embed from home and its constraints might well obscure the psychological consequences of those constraints, such as lack of access to strong networks and inadequate capabilities. Among some Africana persons those deficits has limited their ability to grow in China as opposed to other more well-positioned and skilled individuals. So, while the legacy from home is costly, it can also be a source of the attributes and skills necessary to manage the ambivalence of modernity.

Capitalism, Globalization, and Migration

Given that the overarching objective of capitalists is to increase their base of capital, they forever seek to be as unconstrained as possible in pursuit of opportunities to do so. This can seemingly resonate with the individual's wish to pursue knowledge and wealth with the minimum of limits. Capitalism is therefore entwined with modernity in that it forever seeks new avenues of expression given its essentially insatiable pursuit of greater capital accumulation. Given this impetus, it generates mechanisms and structures that efficiently disseminate the attractiveness of the pursuit and the acquisition of wealth. That feature of globalization is, however, Janus-faced, as it facilitates creative and reflective processes that both favor and question wealth accumulation for its own sake. Many transnational workers and immigrants, initially in thrall of capitalism and intoxicated by its offerings, sometimes become aware of its limits and become at least ambivalent, if not actively opposed, to the challenges that capitalism presents to attempts at holistic self-development, the building of supportive communities, and the maintenance of ethical bulwarks.

Risks

The modern world, with its increasingly globalized systems, offers, through transnational movement, opportunities for self-improvement as well as the risks of being commodified and lonely. In such a world with seemingly infinite options, self-construction can be paradoxically homogenized. This comes about as not all models of self-transformation are equally accessible, nor are all necessarily in the individual's best interests. Walls (2003) argues that one consequence of the model of modern and fairly autonomous individuals is that they can sometimes marginalize the particularity that comes from being located in a specific community, with its moral demands, restrictions, and their ethical obligations to others. This aspect of modernity, which speaks to the obscured influence of neoliberalism, Walls argues, promotes a disingenuous presentation of the self as healthily autonomous, when in reality, it is always at risk for being impoverished and having limited agency.

Capitalism in late modernity is potentially oppressive of the individual through the seduction of consumption that lulls and distracts but does not satiate deeper aspects of being. What is often offered is not a chance to be ethically autonomous but in fact Hobbesian invitations to a narrow worldview that leads to a life focused on consumption and work. Such a shallow but sensuous world constitutes a particular type of risk for the more affluent Africana person in China: the risk of embracing the illusion of a hyper-individuality of unlimited access but often results in individuals feeling that they don't belong anywhere

(Strenger, 2013). Such cosmopolitanism carries the risk of a nuanced anomie given that in its extreme forms it features a lack of commitment to any community with its demands for interdependency, and at times non-reciprocated generosity. In China, I witnessed a small cohort of such individuals; they appear to drift from one host country to another, uneasy, and eternally ambivalent.

Berlant (2011) notes that for those with modest work-related capabilities, embedded in low-resource networks, the outlook can be grim due to their internalization of the myth that despite being low-skilled and under-resourced, they can hold their own in socioeconomic spaces of increasing flux, uncertainty, and crisis. From Berlant's perspective, such individuals are a manifestation of cruel optimism given their hope against all evidence that they can achieve their receding goals for self-development. There are hints of this in elements of the Africana population in China: Some are at a standstill, having failed to achieve skill enhancement or material gain and being unable to generate enough income and the necessary surpluses to exit China as they eventually must (Haugen & Diederich, 2016d). Here, the ambivalence is not adaptive but has a dystopian patina. Individuals who are impoverished and have weak supports are trapped in a China that does not want them; their entrapment is intensified by the fact that they are reluctant to return to a home that cannot support them.

The Multicultural Self

Many Africana persons in Africa, its diaspora, and especially in the Americas have been socialized in multicultural communities, in which there was greater acceptance of a multiplicity of ways to express one's Africana heritage. In many countries, these various assertions of African legacies influenced and were influenced by interactions with other cultural groups. So there is a bias toward transculturalism and regionalism, and such cultures have evolved adaptive ways to manage cultural tensions (Headley, 2011). The experiences of Africana persons make possible a certain degree of epistemological fluidity. This reflects an ongoing attempt to understand what makes one culturally unique alongside an awareness of commonalities with other cultural communities, while not being reduced to some amorphous polyglot (Headley, 2011).

This offers a distinct advantage to Africana persons with migratory tendencies, as they have a history of exposure to that which lies within and between African legacies. They are familiar with commonalities across cultural boundaries and sensitive to differences that are culturally substantive. What might well be a struggle for them, as evidenced by some Africana persons in China, is the value they attach to such differences. So some reported being on one hand motivated and energized by the dynamism of the Chinese, while at the same time bemoaning the cutthroat and at times unethical business culture. Others report a sense of rediscovery and pride in the commonalities they shared with other persons of Africana heritage and at the same time report having been cognizant of substantive differences between them.

The manner in which the Africana individual manages the vicissitudes of self-development in general and its manifestation in a seemingly modernistic and selectively neoliberal China is influenced by how he or she manages developmental urgencies and their attendant pleasures and anxieties. These in turn contribute to the quality of the adaptive style that the Africana person adopts in dealing with the intoxicating and at the same time sobering realities of being in China. Individuals who migrate with a history of being cared for, who are resilient and adept at managing passion and containing disappointment, tend to be relatively successful in China. They are embedded in a healthy and diverse set of relationships, and they are able to eat bitterness but do not flee. They are also fairly adept at managing separation and loss, especially when the goal is to pursue new experiences and self-growth.

Given that most of the individuals I spoke to were under the age of 35 and were university graduates, one could cautiously argue that they are biased to make audacious moves and are not overly preoccupied with concerns around failure or melancholia. For them, modernity represents autonomy and the opportunity to dis-embed from developmentally bleak home settings that generated much ambivalence. These settings, while revered for the intimate attachments, were unacceptable given their structural constraints on spontaneity, risk taking, and intellectual development, and their limited opportunities to generate wealth.

Paradoxically, Africana people in China, who are confronted with being *other*, have the opportunity to resume the lifelong task of understanding their multiplicity of selves in a setting that is often ambivalent toward them. Access to community and the commitment to engage in discourse are feasible in a world that offers the possibility of enquiry, revaluation of the past, and hopefully strategizing about a future self. Being abroad in a world of infinite variants of self offers the Africana person an opportunity to better manage and possibly sequester ways of being that are a legacy of a history of undue constraints and denigration of cultural aspects of identity (Hall, 2002).

The Somewhat Reflective Self

The individual is predisposed to be reflective within a self that can be productively irrational, and such reflective activity is a contingency interacting with and at times muting other contingencies. Such a stance must be well modulated so as to limit the constraints of the influential but often unacknowledged tug of tradition, but not unduly constrain the spontaneities sometimes necessary to exploit uncertainty.

Given that how the individual reflects is influenced by cultural legacies, it was not surprising to observe many Africana persons in China struggling, some fruitfully, to healthily manage their ambivalence. Subjects would often observe that they were not overly reflective about the China they imagined prior to leaving home, as they might have not come given the conservative bias toward launching into the cultural enigma that many home cultures have constructed China to be. Being young and exposed to diverse information sources, many Africana persons chose to leap before looking, assuming that resilience, spontaneity, and an eye for opportunity would stand them in good stead once they arrived in China. Upon arrival, reflective capabilities become more evident among successful Africana workers who negotiate opportunity and risk in a context of uncertainty. This is especially challenging given the stress on a view of modernity in China where the market is the dominant attractor, and the past, while influential, is ambivalently acknowledged.

Modernity and Ambivalence

Modernity has unleased the indulgence of curiosity, privileging individual autonomy and limiting the traditional capacity of the group to overly constrain self-development. This presents the individual who migrates with unprecedented opportunities to discover and develop the self, but given the fluidity of possibilities and the risks of materialistic distractions, unthinking indulgence can result in underdevelopment. It would seem that to both protect and nurture the self, the individual's ambivalence must be managed with the goal of discovering pleasure within reasonable limits in tension with the joys of spontaneity. Given that mindless consumption is a risk in a capitalist-inflected modernity, individuals must manage the temptation of developing a self that is overly attuned to market values and the ever-thirsting for more. They must enjoy the pleasures of consumption but carefully manage the risk of addiction. Again, there is the tension that speaks to ambivalence; given the temptations of an overly materialistic world, a gratification of primordial urges must be in tension with a disciplining of those states.

A state of disciplined curiosity and consumption might be attainable for the Africana person who can reflect on and adaptively manage aspects of the ambivalence-inflected limit that is a legacy from the home country. A too strongly felt sense of ambivalence can make it difficult for the individual to take advantage of opportunities. With healthy group support and adequate reflection, ambivalence can be fruitfully managed as part of the ongoing work of self-development.

References

Adams, C. J. (2014). Afro-Caribbean people in China: Away from home and at home with self. *Caribbean Journal of Psychology*, 6(1), 1–20.

Adams, C. J. (2015). Structure and agency: Africana immigrants in China. *Journal of Pan African Studies*, 7(10), 85–108.

Bauman, Z. (1991). *Modernity and ambivalence*. London, UK: Polity Press.

Bauman, Z. (2001). Identity in the globalizing world. *Social Anthropology*, 9(2), 121–129.

Bauman, Z. (2003). *Liquid love*. London, UK: Polity Press.

Berlant, L. (2011). *Cruel optimism*. Durham, NC: Duke University Press.

Binkley, S. (2011). Psychological life as enterprise: Social practice and the government of neo-liberal interiority. *History of the Human Sciences*, 24(3), 83–102.

Bodnar, S. (2004). Remember where you came from: Dissociative process in multicultural individuals. *Psychoanalytic Dialogues*, 14(5), 581–603.

Bodomo, A. (2012). *Africans in China*. Amherst, NY: Cambria Press.

Castillo, R. (2015). Homing' Guangzhou: Emplacement, belonging and precarity among Africans in China. *International Journal of Cultural Studies*, 18(2), 1–20.

Crouch, C. (2016). *The knowledge corrupters: Hidden consequences of the financial takeover of public life*. Cambridge, UK: Polity Press.

de Haas, H. (2014). Migration theory: Quo vadis? (DEMIG project paper 24, University of Oxford: International Migration Institute).

Freire, P. (2000). *Pedagogy of the oppressed*. New York, NY: Continuum.

Hall, S. (2002). Political belonging in a world of multiple identities. In S. Vertovec & R. Cohen (Eds.), *Conceiving cosmopolitanism: Theory, context and practice* (pp. 25–32). New York, NY: Oxford University Press.

Haugen, H. (2012). Nigerians in China: A second state of immobility. *International Migration*, 50(2), 65–80.

Haugen, H. (2015). Destination China: The country adjusts to its new migration reality. Retrieved from http://migrationpolicy.org/article/destination-china-country-adjusts-its-new-migration-reality

Haugen, H., & Diederich, M. (2016a). Decision to leave home. Retrieved from https://uturnasia.com/2016/01/26/test/

Haugen, H., & Diederich, M. (2016b). From the Gambia to China. Retrieved from https://uturnasia.com/2016/01/25/test11/

Haugen, H., & Diederich, M. (2016c). Life in China. Retrieved from https://uturnasia.com/2016/01/24/test-1/

Haugen, H., & Diederich, M. (2016d). Getting out of China. Retrieved from https://uturnasia.com/2016/01/23/18/

Haugen, H., & Diederich, M. (2016e). Returning home. Retrieved from https://uturnasia.com/2016/01/22/returning-home/

Haugen, H., & Diederich, M. (2016f). Imagining a future. Retrieved from https://uturnasia.com/2016/01/20/aspirations/

Headley, C. (2011). George Lamming and the epistemology of exile: Ways of seeing, singularity and colonialism. In A. Bogues (Ed.), *The George Lamming reader: The aesthetics of decolonialisation* (pp. 287–310). Kingston, Jamaica: Ian Randle Publishers.

Hermans, H., & Dimaggio, G. (2007). Self, identity, and globalization in times of uncertainty: A dialogical analysis. *Review of General Psychology*, 11(1), 31–61.

Joas, H. (2013). *The sacredness of the person: A new genealogy of human rights*. Washington, DC: Georgetown University Press.

Martin, J., & Sugarman, J. (2000). Between the modern and the postmodern: The possibility of self and progressive understanding in psychology. *American Psychologist*, *4*, 397–406.

Matthews, G. (2011). *Ghetto at the center of the world: Chungking mansions.* Chicago, IL: University of Chicago Press.

Pruyser, P. (1983). *The play of the imagination: Toward a psychoanalysis of culture.* New York, NY: International Universities Press.

Rodney, W. (2011). *How Europe underdeveloped Africa.* Baltimore, MD: Black Classic Press.

Senior, O. (2014). *Dying to better themselves: West Indians and the building of the Panama Canal.* Kingston, Jamaica: University of The West Indies Press.

Smart, B. (1999). *Facing modernity: Ambivalence, reflexivity and morality.* London, UK: Sage Publications.

Snow, P. (1988). *The star raft: China's encounter with Africa.* New York, NY: Weidenfeld & Nicholson.

Strenger, C. (2013). The new cosmopolitans: Challenges and discontents. *Psychoanalytic Psychology*, *30*(2), 264–280.

United Nations Department of Economic and Social Affairs Population Division. (2013). The number of international migrants worldwide reaches 232 million. Retrieved from http://esa.un.org/unmigration/documents/The_number_of_international_migrants.pdf

Van Hear, N. (2014). Reconsidering migration and class. *International Migration Review*, *48*(S1), 100–121.

Walls, G. (2003). Toward a critical global analysis. *Psychoanalytic Dialogues*, *14*(5), 605–634.

Wilkerson, I. (2010). *The warmth of other suns.* New York, NY: Vintage Books.

Williams, E. (1994). *Capitalism and slavery.* Durham, NC: University of North Carolina Press.

Wyatt, D. (2009). *The Blacks of premodern China.* Philadelphia, PA: University of Philadelphia Press.

5 Race and Ethnicity

Given China's traumatic experiences at the hands of foreigners, it takes a stance bordering on hostility to cultural difference. It is attracted to the technological innovations of other cultures, especially the West, but it is actively resistant to non-Chinese, and more specifically non-Han cultural diversity. Internally, it is equally vigilant about any cultural strains that challenge the worldview of the majority and dominant Han ethnic group. The goal appears to be to assimilate all other ethnic group into Han culture. Given such a stance, Africana persons are unlikely to be assimilated into mainstream Chinese culture in any significant numbers. For them China is a way station, a temporary home in which to acquire skill, wealth, and experience and then move on.

Cautionary Points in Seeking to Understand Chinese Attitudes to Race and Ethnicity

In seeking to understand the history and contemporary experiences of Africana persons in China, some cautions are necessary. The first of these are that given the limits of contemporary historiography, one must be wary of the assumptions that archivists and historians have made across time, in how they have defined Africa and dark-skinned people (Wyatt, 2009, 2012). In categorizing inter-group differences over time periods, caution must be exercised given the lack of continuity of meaning of how groups are defined. Wyatt (2009, 2012), in his long view on the history of "Blacks" in China going back to the seventh-century, notes that the term *Kunlun* was often ascribed to any dark-skinned person, although such persons did not necessarily come from the space we currently define as Africa. Wyatt (2012) notes that more than likely, they were from current day Indonesia and the Malay Peninsula, as is evident in the passage cited later in this chapter from Spence (1984).

Equal caution should be applied with regard to the interpretive models that they have used to understand the degree of agency that Africans exercised. Such prudence is necessary to avoid unwittingly homogenizing

Africana persons, as Black reflecting a need to buffer against eons old dehumanization pressures (Ademoyo, 2009; Echeruo, 1999) Caution is also necessary in portraying Africana individuals as being fully autonomous and having substantial authority to reimagine themselves and their place in the world (Hall, 1990). Echeruo (1999) argues that the typical Africana person, while experiencing rich subjectivities and striving to be free, is not as unfettered as modernists who privilege autonomous agency would have us believe.

Carefulness is also necessary in discussing features of China in unthoughtful opposition to similar features in the West, with a bias toward marginalizing similarities. There is often the tendency to portray China from the perspective of negative exceptionality, using terms such as xenophobic, closed-minded, and racist or to overstate the power of the state in China by portraying China as stifling all self-expression. Yet at the same time, one can observe an understatement of the role of the market and the attendant resource inequality in the West that also limits individual autonomy and possibility. Here, the challenge is to identify deep commonalities that are obscured by surface differences and also to locate differences that are substantive. So, as Zang (2015) notes, rights regimes in China focus on the interests of the dominant Han group, as opposed to the emphasis in the West on individual rights. This would speak to both a commonality with the West, which has its own racial and ethnic hierarchy, and a substantive difference given the explicit marginalization of individual rights.

Antipathy to Difference

Spence (1984) speaks to long-standing Chinese antipathy toward ethnic difference:

> At the end of that year Ricci and Ruggieri were settled on the edge of Chao-ch'ing city, under the protection of the prefect Wang P'an, who coveted a clock for himself. Since the Jesuits were desperate for funds to complete construction of their first church, Ruggieri went back to Macao to raise money and buy a clock for Wang P'an, which the latter had promised to pay him for handsomely. Finding Macao a desolate place because the Japanese trading ship on which the fortunes of the little colony depended had not arrived, and unable to raise cash to buy a clock for the prefect, Ruggieri had the happy idea of sending the best clockmaker in Macao to join Ricci in Chao-ch'ing. The man, who agreed to the assignment, was "a black from the Canary Islands who had lived in India" ("un Canarino dall'India, di colore assai negro"), according to Ricci. Eager to speed the work, the prefect made available two Chao-ch'ing metal-working craftsmen to assist the Indian. Thus for a

> brief moment in China's history both Chinese and European-trained craftsmen were working by mutual agreement on a technical project under the joint supervision of a Westerner and a Chinese scholar without external or imperial interference. This dramatically suggests a model for the development of universal scientific cooperation, but unfortunately the prefect ordered the Indian back to Macao before the work was finished, after angry Chinese anti-Christians made him the scapegoat in a trumped-up child-harassment case.
>
> (p. 181)

Notable in this passage is the attraction to innovative Western technologies and skills. Themes of the diversity of cultural groups interacting with the Chinese and the resistance to accommodating such diversity are also evident. A subtext to this, as Spence (1990) notes, is the occasional indifference of the Chinese elites to establishing procedures for interacting with foreigners so as to regularize relations. This is a theme reflected in its contemporary immigration policies, which are only now being codified (Castillo, 2016).

China's Conundrum

China seeks to assert itself as a global economic and political power. It has embraced some aspects of the globally dominant neoliberal ethos, and this has transformed its economy into an export behemoth, while at the same time reducing the level of poverty in China, especially among the rural population (Yao, 2000). At the same time, it must grapple with transitioning from a manufacturing and mostly export-oriented economy to one that increasingly generates high-value products for a developing domestic market and a competitive export market. This requires a shift from manufacturing goods often based on Western intellectual creations to production based increasingly on Chinese innovations and aimed at its own growing domestic market. Given the current shortcomings of its educational system, China currently lacks the technical skill base, policy framework, and administrative structures to smoothly make this transition and must rely on Western knowledge and skilled talent from the global marketplace (Wang, H., 2011).

This need to turn to the West engenders much ambivalence on the part of the Chinese given their long-standing antipathy toward the foreigner alongside their attraction to their intellectual resources (Dikotter, 1992; Zang, 2015). In addition, there is a worldwide shortage of skilled personnel, making for fierce competition for their talent. Chinese demand for innovative workers is filled in part by talented and skilled Africana persons, who perceive China as a locale for business opportunities and jobs.

These global and domestic forces have wrought changes on the structure of Chinese society and the quality of agency among its citizens and foreign residents. Skill levels, a sense of individualism, and bounded autonomy are on the rise, and these are crucial ingredients for the creativity and innovation that China requires. These new ways of experiencing the self, are however accompanied by increased demands by citizens for social justice and related rights, a development viewed with antipathy by the state.

China's political directorate perceives these renewed assertions for openness to new ways of thinking, including demands for limits on the authority of the state, as a threat to its ideological hegemony (Hui, 2009). So while Africana persons in China, as skilled foreigners, are beneficiaries of the intellectual and wealth-making opportunities that China offers, they also face official resistance to their attempts to create inclusive and rights-sensitive communities.

Creativity: Systemic Challenges and Obstacles

China has complex and long-standing initiatives to further develop the infrastructure necessary to raise the level of innovation with the aim of transitioning the economy from one based on basic manufacturing to one that generates innovative and high-value products (Wang, H, 2011). Historically however, both external and internal factors have hampered Chinese attempts to unleash its creative energies. The wide distribution of knowledge has always been viewed with ambivalence in China, as while there was an interest in being enlightened and progressing, there was always the fear that such knowledge might prove to be disruptive of the established order (Spence, 1990). The current guarded stance toward the West in China also reflects its painful and instructive memory of predations by foreigners, including the foreign Manchu dynasty (1644–1911), and in the nineteenth and twentieth century, the Japanese, the British, the Germans, and the Americans (Spence, 1990). These foreign-initiated traumatic incursions, which presented challenges to the Han worldview and assaults on its territorial integrity, have heightened the fear of instability and the need for vigilance (Spence, 1990; Zang, 2015).

In its efforts to create a more innovative economy, China must grapple with a host of other challenges. The first of these is the aging of its workforce, which is, in part, a consequence of the one-child policy resulting in a bulge of older workers approaching retirement and a dearth of younger workers given the low reproductive rate in the late twentieth century (Wang, F., 2010). A second source of talent shortage is the wave of anti-intellectualism and the attendant consequences of the shutting down of the university system during the Cultural Revolution during the 1960s. This has resulted in a relative lack of experienced senior managers in current day China (Simon & Cao, 2009).

Even where there is a commitment to a policy of facilitating innovation, the school culture is still mired in memorization and regurgitation of facts, pedagogical approaches that do not promote critical thinking and innovation (Wang, D., 2011). Exacerbating such an approach is Chinese ambivalence toward the West, as it is evident in some policies such as a cautious business school curricula approach with regard to talent management originating in the West. Chinese curricula are found wanting, given their focus on narrowly focused technical skill training, a problem not peculiar to China (Cooke, Saini, & Wang, 2014). This results in an increasing amount of college graduates who lack the creative skill sets necessary to meet China's continued economic growth needs (Simon & Cao, 2009), and given their high unemployment rates, they are a potential source of social unrest (Wang, H., 2011).

Especially challenging has been the creation of a work culture that offers the autonomy that top-flight, foreign-trained talent is used to. In addition is the need to develop oversight mechanisms that ensure that national needs are addressed without unduly impinging on that autonomy that is critical for the creative process and the need for innovative thinking and risk taking. Africana managers in Chinese corporations consistently complain that the extant corporate cultures make it difficult to develop a work ethic that values innovative thinking and risk taking (Adams, 2015).

A particularly daunting challenge in China is the paradox of creativity. Creative thinkers do best in settings that work well with the tension between individual talent and group support. Too much emphasis on individual talent often results in under-productivity, given self-absorption and a reluctance to address group demands. At the same time, an overemphasis on group norms can result in a work culture that stifles creativity. As a consequence, one observes productive mediocrity, a less than adequate performance in terms of the generation of innovative outcomes (Phan et al., 2010).

Related to this paradox is an equally substantive challenge: In promoting creativity and innovation, such individuals do not limit their thoughts to preferred spheres such as the economic and the technical, but also challenge the extant systems in terms of social justice, governance models, and authority relations. This creates a substantive dilemma for the Chinese authorities that are struggling with how best to encourage innovative practices in business and in science and at the same time limit rights demands. This is challenging given that it has historically proven difficult to subordinate the smart and the creative with their fertile and discerning imaginations and their skepticism toward authority and being constrained. It is also challenging as the low productivity can lead to social unrest, which is the overriding fear of China's leaders, given the millions of inadequately prepared university graduates annually seeking jobs. One can observe this challenge play out among a subset of Africana workers in southern China who are successful and are also placing rights demands, albeit modest ones, on the Chinese authorities (Adams, 2015).

With the encouragement of individualism and the shortage of talent, China struggles with low levels of loyalty to the organization, especially by highly skilled individuals who, embedded in a market culture, engage in opportunistic behavior as manifested by frequent job hopping in pursuit of salary and career advancement (Ariga et al., 2012). Many Chinese companies appear to privilege commitment to the company as the most valued attribute of the employee as opposed to the employees' skills and input. They do not view the workplace as a meritocracy, but one that reflects revered relational qualities as paramount (Cooke, Saini, & Wang, 2014). Finally, there are the challenges of developing systems, human resource requirements, and working conditions that reflect China's shift from a planned economy based on manufacturing to a creative economy responsive to market needs that is able to generate innovative processes and products (Wang, H., 2011). Again, some Africana entrepreneurs have proven to be quite adroit at managing this transition going from being exporters to being service providers to being Africana exporters. Others have moved from being suppliers to purchasing manufacturing facilities and designing and producing the greater value-added products that are in demand.

In examining a comparable situation in South Korea, Kim (2009) framed the issue as a tension between ethnic nationalism and civic nationalism. In a globalized marketplace, there is pressure to respect individual rights, and that in turn is crucial to attracting and keeping talent that is in short demand and is attracted to locales that respect individuality. China, in advocating ethnic nationalism, seeks to protect its traditional definition of its national interests, and these interests are not always congruent with a growing, talented, individualized, and culturally diverse middle class or the increasing amount of highly skilled foreign workers in China (Cooke, Saini, & Wang, 2014).

To address some of these challenges, a National Medium- and Long-term Talent Development Plan (2010–2020) was launched. Strategies include recruiting talented individuals from abroad, and in this regard, many Chinese nationals have returned to China to take up senior positions in both academia and business (Wang, H., 2011). Trends that have contributed to the development of the plan include policies in the academic research community reflective of market-oriented approaches to working conditions, with a shift to merit increases and the decline in lifetime appoints in the case of tenure appointments (Suttmeier, Cao, & Simon, 2006).

Recruiting overseas talent through its Thousand Talents initiative has been another tactic China has employed, although it is not capable of completely meeting the national demand for talent (Wang, H., 2011). China has also begun to develop visa regimes supportive of its pursuit of talented individuals. In 2012, China announced the creation of a "talent visa" and in addition has made it relatively easier for talented or affluent foreigners to be eligible for permanent residency visas (Haugen, 2015). Such an influx of talent, however, also means an influx of ideas about how China should evolve and a concomitant questioning of the systems necessary to facilitate and sustain such development. These issues raise the question of China's historical and contemporary attitude toward difference with a focus on ethnicity, race, and the foreigner.

China's Han-Centric Worldview

The historical ambivalence of the dominant Han ethnic group in China toward cultural difference in general is manifested in its wariness of the foreigner, the Black, and its own minority ethnic groups (Dikotter, 1992; Zang, 2015).

China has historically constructed a worldview that placed China and its perceptions as paramount. So, curiosity about the world is tempered by a sense of superiority and a long-standing mistrust, wariness, and at times withdrawal (Spence, 1990). This somewhat jaundiced worldview is due in large part to the experiences of the dominant Han group with its history of long periods of subjugation to ethnic groups such as the Manchus and to external powers such as the French, British, Japanese, Dutch, and Americans (Mitter, 2004). There is an ambivalent quality to this stance: The dominant Han ethnic group values China's uniqueness and is vigilant with regard to both its territorial integrity and ideological hegemony, but it is also quite attuned to some aspects of what it needs to learn from other cultures especially with regard to technology and also in terms of how to maintain its authority and that of the Communist Party of China (CPC). In this regard, it is worth noting that the Han ethnic group and the CPC are both routinely conflated to embody the Chinese state. Being a strong international power is essential to China's view of itself as a reemerging superpower attuned to its economic and security interests and determined to have its perspectives respected by the international community (Baijia, 2009; Fallows, 2016).

Consistent with such a Sino-centric worldview has been the Chinese historical attitude toward non-Chinese persons, expressed often as a tendency to establish hierarchies of "barbarians" in which those with dark complexions occupied the lowest intellectual and civilized rung (Dikotter, 1992). The belief was that China "was the 'central' kingdom and that other countries were, by definition, peripheral, removed from the center of the universe" (Spence, 1990, p. 119). A prominent feature of the Chinese attitude to the foreigner was therefore one of disparagement, a view of them as inferior, but at the same time, there was a notable vigilance, given the foreigners' business savvy and their technological prowess.

According to Spence (1990), intermarriage, alliances, and measured tolerance were all deployed to maintain China's enduring quest for harmony and stability. Although trade during the eighteenth and nineteenth centuries was a means of maintaining harmony, it was permitted from a perspective of tribute paying, a demanded acknowledgement of the superiority of the Chinese in relation to its neighbors (Spence, 1990). As is still currently the case, while trading was tolerated, temporary residences for traders were segregated, and permanent residency was discouraged.

Given China's intermittent lack of nuanced curiosity about the diversity of foreigners, it is not easy to tease out African peoples from among the many dark-skinned ethnic groups that have inhabited Asia and that interacted with China (Jayasuriya, 2006). What little exposure the Chinese have had to dark-skinned persons came mostly in the form of enslaved persons (Dikotter, 1992). Again, however, one observes the ambivalence toward *other*, as while there is an historical antipathy toward the foreigner and the non-Han groups, there is also a keen appreciation of the skills and knowledge sets that otherwise "inferior" groups possess that could be useful to China in its quest to be a dominant and respected power.

So, there is a persistent interest in foreign talent, technology, and innovative practices to the degree that the foreigner can enhance creativity and productivity, facilitate domestic stability, bolster the hegemony of the ruling elites, and burnish China's international reputation (Zang, 2015). This sits alongside a questionable assumption that these imported ways of being in the world will not in subtle ways change China's perception of itself as non-Western. The hope is that despite the intellectual and cultural imports, they would be able to maintain their focus on purity and to resist Western ideas of individuality, hybridity, and cultural diversity (Dikotter, 1992; Zang, 2015).

Subjugation and the Wariness Toward the Foreigner

Globalized capitalism, driven by the goods-seeking and subjugation policies of the incipient European colonial powers from the sixteenth century on challenged China's indifference to matters foreign and its view of itself as superior. At first, the Chinese forced the initial British traders, with their interest in tea, porcelain, and textiles, to accept the tributary system with its high fees, limited access, and administrative red tape (Spence, 1990). This created a significant trade imbalance to the favor of the Chinese, who demonstrated scant interest in importing European goods.

The solution to this payment imbalance was a triangular trade that saw British goods exported to India, where the profits were used to purchase opium from British-controlled India, which was then exported to

China. The earnings from this would pay for British-bought Chinese goods destined for the European market that received significant markups in price on each leg of the transaction (Spence, 1990). The social and health impacts of heroin imports were devastating, resulting in widespread addiction, human suffering, and the social instability and corruption that flow from drug trafficking and substance abuse. The Chinese perceived this Western-driven toxicity, over time, to be consistent with their view of foreigners as barbarians bent on undermining their sovereignty, a motif very much present in contemporary Chinese perception of foreign powers (Fallows, 2016).

These and similar impositions by the West and by Japan were also perceived as an attempt to subordinate Chinese values to those of their foreign antagonists, a move that was and continues to be resisted by the Chinese (Mitter, 2004; Spence, 1990; Zang, 2015).

These impositions included mandated Western imports, administrative structures, and tax regimes, as well as engaging in outright warfare, all of which the Chinese resisted at great cost. The common thread was a sense of a lack of respect for Chinese sovereignty and its right to develop its own worldview and practices (Mitter, 2004; Spence, 1990). This is a theme that is quite resonant in contemporary China with its marked ambivalence toward the West. On one hand, China is engaged in a quest for Western technology and innovative cultural practices and, on the other hand, resists its pressure for generous trade conditions, cultural diversity, individual rights, and Western style democracy (Fallows, 2016; Zang, 2015).

Ethnicity Within China: Ronghe—The Elimination of Substantive Ethnic Diversity

Zang (2015), in his comprehensive account of ethnicity within China, argues that the ultimate goal of the Han majority group is to acculturate and assimilate over time all other ethnic groups into a Han worldview and lifestyle. This would gradually lead to a decline in substantive ethnic diversity. So, while otherness has existed within China for centuries, manifested as within-Han and between-Han differences, the long-term aim is to significantly reduce such otherness. The ambivalence toward otherness is evident through the promotion of non-threatening aspects of ethnicities and affirmative action programs. This is in uneasy coexistence with hierarchies of ethnicity, denigration of some ethnic practices, and the ever-present push for assimilation:

> The determining factor in Beijing's attitude towards an ethnic minority group is its political inclination: the minority nationalities that are willing to accept state control and the official depiction of their ethnic group and histories have been treated favorably. Beijing is more

> willing to grant them some freedom to exercise their lawful rights, practice their cultures and religions and join CCP and government ranks. The minority nationality groups such as Tibetans and Uyghurs that have demanded more control over their identities, more autonomy, or even independence have regularly been confronted with government repression.
>
> (Zang, p. 124)

At the same time, such willingness to adopt the government's narrative of the group's identity leads to increasing acculturation and eventually yields assimilation and the disappearance of substantial aspects of the group's original culture.

Zang (2015) highlights the policy of *ronghe* as a manifestation of the eventual elimination of substantive ethnic and cultural diversity. Historically, as a consequence of the Han ethnic group expanding by assimilating the groups it conquered, such groups would lose their unique cultural identity and adopt the language, customs, and worldview of the Han culture. This speaks to a fusion of the Han and minorities in accordance with Confucian cultural diffusion. *Ronghe* drives acculturation and eventually assimilation as it is antagonistic toward self-determination and substantive cultural diversity. So, the aim is not to create a multi-ethnic society where there is substantive accommodation to culture difference with concomitant authority, where such accommodations would be a threat to the dominance of the Han and, by extension, to that of the Chinese state.

Over time, acculturation was pursued at the cost of respect for cultural difference but with the promise of socioeconomic improvement. The political approach was to portray the non-Han groups as exploited, victims of a class struggle that left them economically inferior to the Han people, so that acculturation would seem to be an attractive option for them. Socioeconomic equality was the promise offered to non-Han people to entice them into assimilation, as opposed to Soviet-like attempts to use force to eliminate other cultures (Zang, 2015). This shifted during the Cultural Revolution, when there were sustained attacks on cultural difference and an insistence on assimilation—on a unified Han China. While the aggression has been muted, the emphasis in contemporary China has been on a process of acculturation that will lead to a degree of assimilation that will eliminate ethnic diversity.

Zang (2015) argues that the dominant Han group thinks such an approach, with its hostility to otherness, reflects sound Confucian principles, given the perception of different ethnic groups as barbarians. It also speaks to a paternalistic ethos that informs China's approach to governance in general and ethnic relations in particular, giving rise to the goal of acculturation into the Han ethnic group and an eventual reduction of cultural diversity. Such a Confucian-infused approach will appear to tolerate, if not celebrate, diversity, but the long-term objective is assimilation. Historically, this approach has had some successes, with other ethnic groups assimilating into Han culture and their own indigenous culture practices atrophying. Chinese nationalism, a relatively recent concept from the nineteenth century, rests on a Han/Confucian base of a homogeneous culture that is stable and harmonious.

Zang (2015) also argues that the privileging of the Han and conflating it with Chinese-ness was troubling to some elements of non-Han ethnic groups, such as the Uyghurs and the Tibetans. These groups do not perceive themselves as part of the emerging creation of a homogenized and pacified China and therefore resist its assimilationist policies. Given the appearance of an advocacy of toleration alongside a goal of acculturation, such policies speak to the strategy of the Han of eliminating substantive difference.

There are 56 official ethnic groups in China of which the Han is the largest (91.8%). Otherness is also reflected in China's sizable population of internal migrants, which is comprised mostly of rural workers moving to urban centers on the east coast (Davin, 2009; Myers, Xiaoyan, & Cruz, 2013; Taylor, 2011). One should add to this the small but growing presence of foreigners including those of Africana heritage.

Many of the 55 minority groups have rich economic resources and are in politically sensitive border areas, so stability is therefore important in these areas. The current system of classification and recognition came out of a desire to create a broadly representative national body that would validate the rule of the CPC. The formal definition of ethnic groups was encoded by the CPC as a means of establishing its legitimacy and that of the state. This required a streamlining process that made administrative decisions regarding what constituted an ethnic group. This resulted in the Ethnic Classification Process of 1953, creating initially 38 groups expanded eventually to the current 56 groups from an original list of over 400, some with as few as one member (Zang, 2015). Han ascendancy has been long in the making, going as far back as 206 BC with setbacks as other groups, often perceived as barbarians, have ruled China, culminating in the Manchu dynasty that ruled China from 1644 to 1911. So, there have always been noticeable ethnic differences within China, alongside a history of perceiving non-Han groups as a threat, with this us/them dynamic not being unique to China. Tapp (in Zang, 2015, pp. 131–132) cautions against creating strict Han/other dichotomies given the growing evidence of fluidity of boundaries between groups, permissiveness of ethnic definitions, and the creation of hybridities and nuanced identifications.

Often, the differences between the minority groups and the Han are quite shallow, leading to assimilation or "ethnicity-lite," as is the case with China's three largest ethnic minority groups, the Zhuang, the Hui, and the Manchu; each of these groups is fairly acculturated into the Han culture with significant loss of indigenous language skills and high intermarriage rates into the Han group (Zang, 2015). By contrast, in the case of other groups, cultural differences are quite pronounced and often adversarial, such as the relationships between the Han, and the Tibetans, and the Uyghurs.

The administrative defining and ordering of ethnic groups often obscures marked within group differences, with elements of some groups such as the Uyghurs appearing to become more acculturated in Han ways of being, while other elements are highly resistant. Within groups, one will often observe stratification driven by market conditions and the degree to which members have the capabilities to succeed in a Han-dominated culture. So, issues such as Mandarin language competencies and adopting Han cultural practices become crucial facilitators of success as opposed to a Han-renouncing stance. In this context, affirmative action policies have as a goal integrating their recipients into the dominant Han culture and its worldview; this offer creating divisions within the ethnic group (Zang, 2015).

Going back as far as 202 BC, under the Han dynasty, China has promulgated various policies to acknowledge ethnic diversity and grant some semblance of autonomy in the larger interest of inter-group harmony (Yuan, 2008). In China, the Han-dominated authorities are vigilant to any type of substantive cultural difference, and they pay special attention to ethnic-based assertion of a demand for rights. A given group's threat level is assessed "in terms of numerical strength, geographic concentration, and nationalistic aspirations" (Zang, 2015, p. 126). This can lead to a paradoxical situation in which an ethnic group perceived as a threat is granted more concessions than a group perceived as benign, with such a decision being mediated by what the state believes best serves its interest in terms of stability and territorial integrity among other factors. The concessions are always aimed at promoting acculturation and often result in creating within group divisions, as is the case with the Uyghurs. This approach allows for repression of the splittists—those Uyghurs who wish independence from China—and concessions and benefits to those Uyghurs who seek to acculturate and accept the state's narrative as to the idea of Uyghurs being a part of the Chinese state (Zang, 2015).

Within the Western aggregation of nations, policies have evolved over the past 25 years to a point where minority groups have rights, and the state is held responsible for enforcing and protecting those rights. Koenig (in Zang, 2015) notes that "States are no longer expected to represent a homogeneous national community, but rather have to publically recognize a variety of particularistic collective identities legitimated by universalistic human rights" (p. 174). Chinese government policy seems ambivalent about this approach. An interesting wrinkle on this otherness has been the tendency of some members of the Han to claim minority status so as to recover lost cultural heritage given the permeable boundary between the Han and some minority groups. However, this was also a way for some individuals to avail themselves of affirmative action benefits, which led to an increase in the amount of minority group members relative to the Han majority grouping (Zang, 2015).

Another consequence of affirmative action includes preferential admission to universities as well as to the CPC. The political directorate ensures that within the CPC there is a cultivation of the elites of certain minority groups whose loyalty is to the state, and there is a well-thought-out approach to managing such minority groups. Despite these varied efforts that have raised millions from poverty, there is a marked inequality between the educational and economic outcomes of members of the Han group compared to members of the minority groups; this inequality is also noticeable between members of different minority groups and also between members of the same minority group (Zang, 2015). This raises questions as the availability of resources and equality of access to those resources.

Despite some positive changes, China has adhered to policies that in substance are consistent with acculturation and assimilation:

> Beijing has maintained its policy toward national minorities in China by insisting on the supremacy of state sovereignty and territorial integrity over individual rights and collective minority guarantees. It has defined nationality issues strictly as part of its internal affairs that are not subject to foreign criticism.
>
> (Zang, 2015, p. 186)

The Chinese, as do many other nations, privilege territorial integrity, political stability, and economic growth over individual and minority rights. Over time, as China becomes more integrated into the international community, *ronghe* approaches may prove irrelevant. The Han people may shift their focus to individual liberty and well-being and may have less interest in Han group dominance.

Blackness Construction

For the Chinese, Blackness was not historically essentialized as meaning out of Africa or peculiar to those with Black pigment, but it could also refer to any group perceived as ignorant. The negative ascriptions to a more specific Blackness linked to Africa speaks, in part, to the historical influence of White Western expatriates in China, with their articulation of social Darwinism and negatively essentializing constructions of Africana peoples (Dikotter, 1992). These influential foreigners that included priests and teachers extolled the virtues of Western modes of learning and production, which they linked to racist notions of a superior White "race" that had evolved in contrast to an inferior Black "race."

Fennell (2013) notes that the Chinese thirst for knowledge meant that it was not immune to the essentialized racism embedded in the enlightenment thinking of the West. Such thinking was inextricably linked to Western scientific classification, which some Chinese people venerated, but others questioned (Spence, 1990). Social Darwinism as a manifestation of racialist scientific thinking was used to justify the inferior outcomes of subordinated persons of color. This misuse of Darwin was in the context of attempts by Chinese elites to understand what made the West technologically superior to China. Here, Darwin's thinking was misinterpreted to mean that race-based competition would result in the best group succeeding, assuming that such a group was homogeneous and was united in purpose (Spence, 1990).

Some of the Chinese elites made the erroneous assumption that the superiority of the White race had a genetic basis. The reality of their economic exploitation of persons of color, and the denying to them of fair access to resources to develop their capabilities, did not factor into their understanding of how White superiority was achieved. At the same time, Spence (1990) noted that other Chinese thinkers such as Yan Fu, who had been initially attracted to social Darwinism, began to question its utility. Spence (1990) makes reference to this in his comments about Yan Sun, a leading proponent of such thinking:

> But by 1913, Sun was writing sadly of a world dominated by struggles for survival from which no government or industrial enterprise could be exempt. Yan Fu too, lost his enthusiasm for the theories he had helped so much to popularize in China, writing that the failures of the Chinese republic and the bloodshed of World War I in Europe showed that, (in Yan's words), three hundred years of evolutionary progress have all come down to nothing but four words: selfishness, slaughter, shamelessness, and corruption.
>
> (p. 302)

Fennell (2013) also notes that one lesson that the Chinese Han people took from their long subordination to the Manchus was a rejection of any cultural difference within their ranks. This fear of subordination, foreign domination, and cultural pollution by the other is one that still resonates in contemporary Chinese culture. It coexists uneasily with an awareness of the creative and technological skills of non-Chinese groups and a wish to access and exploit such skills for the task of nation building and the continued hegemony of the Han people.

With the advent of the People's Republic of China (PRC) in 1950, there continued to be a stress on a unified ethnic nation, but there was a beginning nurturance of the idea of ideological solidarity with peoples of other nations. This sense of solidarity would emphasize the commonality of the historical exploitation of China and of peoples of color by the imperialistic and capitalist West (Fennell, 2013). One of the many consequences of this policy was a sense of solidarity with and support for the colonized peoples of Africa and its diaspora in their struggles for freedom. This resonated strongly with China's own struggles for political autonomy in relation to the West. Such solidarity was expressed as a stressing of the similarities between the civilizations of Africa and China, including the challenges they faced in terms of development. This sense of solidarity was also extended to African Americans, and W.E.B. Du Bois was a revered figure in China and made three trips there as an honored guest of the CPC. Such identification was also accompanied by technical assistance, loans, and student scholarships to other developing countries (Fennell, 2013).

Fennell (2013) also noted a particular permutation in the Chinese contemporary use of Blackness, in which they did not essentialize a close association between darkness of skin color and lack of intelligence in people of Africana heritage. This is a critical distinction that becomes evident in twenty-first-century China, where one observes an initial equating of Blackness and ignorance and by extension low *suzhi*, a Chinese term that approximately means the quality of human capabilities (Hairong, 2003). Many Africana workers in China observe that these associations are often somewhat decoupled when many Chinese people do business with them, which typically results in a Chinese acknowledgement of the Africana person as intelligent and astute businesspersons and intellectuals in possession of high *suzhi* (Adams, 2014).

China's decision to selectively adopt global market norms and business practices forces it to confront and modify, but not necessarily renounce, their traditional wariness toward those who are not Han Chinese (Haimei, 2011). Such an approach would be in the service of adopting a sense of civic nationalism that is relatively inclusive but is linked to the ultimate goal of assimilation (Kim, 2009). Despite such progressive thinking and policies, intimations of social Darwinism still informed the thinking if not the actions of some Chinese elites and many of its citizens. There was a sense echoed by others that the Chinese felt inherently superior to the Blacks. As more Black students studied in China, there were tensions and at times riots over issues such as interracial dating and racial profiling by the police and immigration authorities (Hevi, 1962).

These ambivalences continue to be manifested in China around difference in general and race specifically. The embracing of Lou Jing, an Afro-Chinese woman, by some as being part of the ethnic mosaic of China and her vociferous rejection by others due to her difference (Anonymous, 2009a, 2009b) is illustrative. This is also evident in the airing of advertisements widely viewed as racist that speak to ongoing struggles to relinquish racist tropes, and wariness toward difference in general and the foreigner specifically (Castillo, 2016).

Vignette: Lou Jing: Afro-Chinese

Please note that the following vignette differs significantly from the others in this book in that this is the only vignette to feature someone I did not interview personally. Lou Jing was contacted but declined to be interviewed. The data used was extracted from internet sources. I nevertheless chose to use this format because it is a specific situation someone experienced that raises the issues I want to look at in this chapter.

Lou Jing's appearance on Chinese national television as a finalist in the talent show *Go! Oriental Angels* elicited strong positive and negative responses, phenomena not unlike that reported by foreign Africana persons in China. Born in 1989, she is the child of a Chinese mother, Sun Min, and an African American father who left China apparently unaware that he had conceived a child, and whom she has never met. Lou Jing appears to veer between indifference and a sense of loss, not unlike other children in similar situations (Anonymous, 2009a).

There were many harsh judgments against the mother, in part based on the allegation that she was married and had an affair with the African American man, resulting in the pregnancy. One argument seems to be that the mother should be ashamed of having a child out of wedlock or as a result of an affair; some felt that given such shame, she should have not appeared on national television to make manifest the outcome of her immoral behavior, a shame that is extended to the daughter. Others were supportive of the mother, given that she chose to give birth rather than have an abortion.

One of Lou Jing's nicknames was Gong, which means stupid, and Little Black (Anonymous, 2009a). While neither she nor her classmates were bothered by using the name Little Black and denied it had any racial connotations, they objected to non-classmates referring to her that way. Jing portrays herself as being encouraged to be kind to others, and so while bothered by hurtful racialized comments, reportedly tends not to get angry at those making such comments:

> Normally, when I go out, occasionally other people would say something, most of them with good intentions. But there are people with not so good intentions, they would insult me. But just a few words, I listen to them and let it pass. I think it's just annoying, as long as people around me all are very good to me and that is enough.
>
> (Anonymous, 2009a)

Many online respondents to Lou Jing's story struggled with the idea that Jing could be Black and Chinese, while for others, it was not an issue

(Anonymous, 2009b). Some noted that American culture is not sensitive to biracial approaches and that she would be considered Black there. There was difficulty accepting that this Chinese woman with Africana heritage could be fully Chinese and speak Mandarin, given that she is Black. The combination of having a sexual liaison with a foreigner and with one who is Black is also thought to have fueled the rage at her mother and by extension at Lou Jing. Negatives tropes about Black male sexuality were a prominent subtext in some of the comments. Zhou (2009), notes that the negative perception of Blackness reflects a Chinese preference for paleness, given its association for being affluent enough to being able to avoid doing low status outdoor manual labor.

A statement appeared online that people referred to as the Four Pronouncements; it was attributed to Jing, who denied writing the statement (Anonymous, 2009b). The statement reads as follows:

1. My father is an American, not African.
2. I am a native Shanghainese.
3. Parents' fault I should not be responsible for, I am innocent!
4. Solemnly Protest against acts of racial discrimination by some of you, my skin color should not be the target of attacks! I will retain the right to take legal actions!

(Anonymous, 2009b)

As Zhou (2009) also notes, the Four Pronouncements statement reveals a racial hierarchy with regard to the Africana world that others have commented on, where African American is held in higher regard than African. Zhou also observes that many Chinese are unaware of their own issues around colorism, given the range of skin hues to be found in China. It has also been noted that had her father been White, she would have been viewed in a very positive light, given what would be her paleness and the admiration of a White aesthetic in China (Washington, 2009).

This incident is illustrative of China's coming of age in a globalized world with increased inflows of foreigners and ways of thinking about diversity that challenge long-standing and unexamined notions of racial, ethnic, and national purity. Issues around sexuality are also being challenged (Anonymous, 2013). The ensuing debates, while painful at times also reveal nuanced and conflictual positions that challenge the myth of China being a homogeneous society.

Notable in this online debate was the mention of ethnic diversity in China. This was positioned as not simply the difference between the Han majority and the 55 officially acknowledged minority ethnic groups but also within-Han diversity as well such as diversity by region, accent, and skin color. What is difficult to speak definitively about is the distinction between ways of explaining difference based on xenophobia, race, or colorism. Complicating this analysis are the many meanings that could be attributed to Lou Jing's Blackness, including assertions by some that the negative comments may speak to colorism and the favoring of Whiteness as opposed to racism and the denigration of her Blackness. As China must increasingly embrace diversity, if only to be more creative and productive, these issues will continue to demand thoughtful engagement.

Attempts to interpret between group and within group difference in China must be done tentatively, as the imposition of Western analytical forms of analysis might well obscure and distort the issues being examined (Crossley, 1990; Zang, 2015). Often missing from this analysis is a sense of the dynamic and diverse set of groupings that constituted China and interacted with it. Morais' (2009) analysis of Africana persons' centuries-long presence in Macau is an illustration of such a relationship that until recently was not well known.

In summary, this ambivalence toward the Africana person is grounded in a historical antipathy toward foreigners alongside an attraction to their skills. Given the linking of respect and admiration to those who are skilled irrespective of their ethnicity, the Chinese have historically adapted, with mixed feelings and policies, to those who are knowledgeable albeit foreign. This admiration is always in tension with a favoring of a mythically homogeneous and harmonious China, a view under constant pressure as China becomes more exposed to a globalized world with its diverse cultures. As a function of these pressures, China will continue to wrestle with how to embrace difference that is truly different and yet still maintain a seemingly culturally purist sense of what it means to be Chinese.

The seemingly contradictory nature of the goals speaks to China's longstanding fear of instability, territorial fragility, and the decline of the influence of the Han and by extension the Chinese nation. In that regard, Africana persons in China are one embodiment of the ambivalence with which China struggles, because they constitute a promise to enhance China's quest to be creative and tolerant. They also however constitute a threat to China's desires to be a culturally homogeneous society.

Structure, Agency, and Otherness in China

All cultures generate structures that both facilitate and constrain the individual's sense of agency, and over time, that structure is influenced by the agency of its individual members and the groups in which they are embedded. In a previous article (Adams, 2015), based on Sewell's (1992) work, I defined structure as follows: "Structure speaks to a set of schemas or ways of thinking that facilitate or constrain social actions" (p. 87). Traditions, ideologies, policies, and laws all speak to influential schemas that guide social action and are not necessarily conscious (Sewell, 1992). So, in China, the thirst for knowledge has a long history of being in tension with the fear that such knowledge might destabilize hierarchy and order (Spence, 1990).

At the same time, a given structure is comprised of relationships between a diverse set of stakeholders with often differing schemas and access to resources (Bakewell, 2010). Some are in comity and others in tension with each other as a result of competing schemas or differing interpretations of a given schema. So, China's ethnic diversity is a constant source of tension within a structure where the dominant Han ethnic group appears committed, through assimilation, to eliminate ethnic diversity over time; such a strategy being fiercely resisted by some ethnic groups such as the Uyghurs and the Tibetans (Zang, 2015). Structures, therefore, do not faithfully and automatically reproduce as they are subject to contingencies such as the actions of various actors within the system, thereby generating change (Sewell, 1992).

So, for example, some members of minority ethnic groups will choose to appear to acculturate in ways consistent with Han culture so as to access the benefits that come with being identified with that group. Conversely, others who identify as Han, given a context of permeable boundaries with non-Han ethnic groups, will appear to identify with non-Han ethnic groups so as to access affirmative action opportunities (Zang, 2015). This is also evident in the contrasting administrative stance toward Africana merchants in Guangzhou as against Yiwu. In the former, Africana workers portray the authorities as watchful and often hostile to their presence, tending not to promulgate business-friendly policies that are of benefit to the Africana entrepreneur (Bodomo, 2012). In Yiwu, a growing commercial hub, policies are business-friendly, and the authorities there work with Africana businesspersons to nurture and sustain mutually beneficial business relationships (Cisse, 2015).

The Yiwu arrangement is consistent with de Haas' (2014) emphasis on the relational nature of structure and the constraints and possibility for agency that are often negotiated within a pattern of structured relationships. The degree of agency exercised is invariably reflective of the power the individual or group has to influence the decision making that regulates constraints and permissions within the relationship. In that context, China has to a significant degree embraced aspects of a neoliberal ethos as part of its strategy of promoting accelerated rates of economic growth. This embrace has had profound structural effects in terms of the role of the state, economic outcomes, and ways of thinking about the self. One feature of this ethos includes an emphasis on the individual as an autonomous and skilled entrepreneur. Such individuals ideally define themselves in terms of their market value, measured by their ability to generate wealth, and are wary of tradition, the group, and the state (Binkley, 2011; Foster, 2016).

Consistent with a neoliberal ethos, the Chinese state is selective in embracing welfare functions. To its credit, it has moved untold millions out of abject poverty through the provision of better health care, education, housing, and other facilitating structures (Yao, 2000). Alongside this has been an emphasis on wealth generation, and individuals have been encouraged to focus on being financially independent of the state. The expectation is that the individual will take increased responsibility for social duties that since the advent of a communist regime in 1949 were thought of as the responsibility of the state (Kleinman et al., 2011). So, even as China invests more in social services, it is to facilitate the creation of citizens who through their adoption of entrepreneurship will generate the surplus necessary to privately meet their own welfare needs and increasingly that of their aging parents.

As a consequence of this retreat by the state, and the emphasis on individual agency, there is the risk of marginalizing the interdependencies and caring that establish social trust and are the basis of community. The retreat of the state is accompanied by a continued emphasis on surveillance and constraints, where the aim of such a focus is to protect its interests. Such an approach is consistent with a neoliberal ethos, but an inevitable consequence is that elements of the community are increasingly chafing at constraints imposed by the state and are pressing for structures that support a model of self-development that is not limited to wealth generation as a goal in of itself (Binkley, 2011; Freire, 2000).

There are aspects of Chinese culture that reflect the tension between the benefits of modernity and a critique of its risks. This is captured in Kleinman et al.'s (2011) description of Huang Yongyu's (1973) Maoist era painting of an owl with one eye open and the other closed. The open eye can be said to represent awareness and guarded interest in the rush of modernity with its accompanying uncertainty, risk, and opportunity. It also looks unblinkingly to the disruptive technologies, the suffocating bureaucracy, and the challenges of family and work, all in the overall context of being in what Kleinman et al. (2011) refer to as "the blooming buzzing world" (p. 23). The closed eye becomes a metaphor for a removal from immediacy as well as from the cacophony of stimuli and the anxieties and desires that they provoke. It represents a chance to be more reflective and to focus on interdependencies that include but are not limited to family. It speaks to the possibility of constraining the shallow and ultimately narcissistic and dystopian view of a world centered on an almost autistic notion of self. It entertains the possibility of a life committed to and contributing to the well-being of others.

One of the challenges of such introspection is re-acquaintance with sorrow and loss in terms of a keenly felt history of unethical constraints. Kleinman et al. (2011) go on to note that there is an irreducible tension between these two perspectives. This is embodied in the professional life of an Africana worker in Shanghai who asked not to be identified. She portrays herself as being very good at her work as a senior manager and is respected by her Chinese and expatriate peers. A font of ideas, she constantly challenges the business status quo even as she is sensitive to the known but unstated limits:

> I must invite my peers and especially my bosses to entertain possibilities that I damn well know are best for the company, but I cannot go full speed ahead as I would in the [United] States. I must devote much more resources here to building consensus and appearing to defer to the age and the illusion of the wisdom of my bosses. So I find I spent a lot of time contemplating how to act and I am discovering, almost accidentally, new things about myself.

This neoliberal push, consistent with Bauman's (1991) take on modernity, solves some problems and is the midwife of other problems. The state in general and the Chinese state in particular is loath to relinquish its regulatory and constraining capacity, especially in the political realm, and yet must concede some of that authority to globalized market forces. That in turn confronts it with another trade-off in the economic forces it has unleashed over the past 30 years. Its exhortation to its citizens to embrace the market has resulted in the creation of an enlightened middle class that questions the right of the state to be unduly restrictive of its human rights. So, an unintended effect of the pursuit of increased productivity is an increased demand for rights in a culture where the elites are always concerned about its restless citizens and social instability. Historically, the restlessness sprung from hunger and unemployment; now, it might arise from limits on autonomy and on the pursuit of authenticity. Such demands constitute a limit on governmental authority given the power of these groups as relatively autonomous and skilled, as well as crucial to meeting the demands of the market.

A neoliberal market thrives on seemingly autonomous individuals taking chances and bearing the consequences of those actions. It seeks to channel those creative impulses into material consumption as a solution to the individualistic search for authenticity and other meaningful psychological experiences (Binkley, 2011). An unintended effect of such courting of the psyche is the inclination among some to question the nuanced enslavement and narrowness of experiences that come with being embedded in an overly market-oriented culture. This is especially a challenge in China, where the pursuit of the artistic and the spiritual often generates a skeptical and questioning stance on the part of citizen practitioners toward the state. It reveals the hidden hand of control that is part and parcel of the neoliberal ethos, and in China, can often result in a severe restriction on such activities.

In addition to its concerns about its ability to constrain its own population, China must deal with another aspect of its talent conundrum. To compete in an increasingly global marketplace, it must have talented and skilled workers, a group in short supply in China. It must therefore import and at the same time domestically develop such talent, while managing the ambivalence and risks that this generates. The successful pursuit of such talent is essential to China maintaining a competitive posture in the global marketplace. At the same time, the state is wary of the foreigner or the domestic *other* as conduits of ideas that might challenge existing ideologies of control; such challenges would in turn be a threat to the conservative and controlling ethos of the governing elite. Some of these workers are distinctly foreigners such as those from Africa and its diaspora; others are Chinese citizens who have studied abroad and returned to China or were educated in China. All three groups are the purveyors of ways of thinking that are highly desired and also carry a stance toward autonomy and equality that is not as welcomed.

Self-Construction and the Market in China: Human Capabilities and National Development

The Africana person in China is embedded in an environment in the midst of rapid change but still profoundly influenced by long-standing cultural attitudes toward the pursuit of status and the need for stoicism or the eating of bitterness. At the same time, there is a healthy, expanded sense of agency relative to what was possible in the home country. This coexists alongside an awareness of considerable and specific social constraints on selective areas of personal growth.

It is difficult to identify any one dominant ideology in China. Its government is clearly authoritarian, given the severe limits it places on individual rights and the relatively modest influence that its citizenry has over the activities of the ruling CPC (Griffiths & Zeuthen, 2014). In addition, ancient epistemologies that are no longer politically privileged continue to deeply influence Chinese ways of thinking and acting. One such tendency noted earlier is ambivalence around the democratization of knowledge manifested as a relative openness to knowledge but a marked wariness with regard to the underlying autonomy promoting epistemologies that accompany such knowledge. This age-old concern of China's elites is that these perspectives might undermine their authority, so the proponents of substantive difference must be carefully policed. This stance has created a daunting dilemma for China given its increasing integration into the world economy and the ideas and challenges that this presents to a culture that values control and the sequestering of knowledge.

China has adopted certain elements of a neoliberal approach to help guide the country's management of human market-oriented development and economic progress. This includes a neoliberal focus among certain elites on economic prosperity rather than individual progress in the area of agency and rights. This speaks to ideological uncertainty and confusion, as the goal is for individuals to attain a certain level of status that differentiate them from others in the lower economic strata, an idea that contradicts Marxist notions of an increasingly homogeneous society (Anagnost, 2004). This differentiation is based on the quality of one's knowledge or *suzhi that is informed in ways that are not always clear such as the individual's geographical location and family lineage.* The term *suzhi*, discussed below, is a complex Chinese concept that lacks an English language equivalent and speaks to class standing, cognitive skill sets, and status markers such as the political credentials of one's parents, among others (Hairong, 2003; Kipnis, 2007).

Suzhi: Self-Improvement

It is quite difficult to articulate a definitive sense of the Chinese term *suzhi*. It generally speaks to an embodied quality, with an emphasis on cognition and the acquired skill sets that are especially attractive to the market. It has many variants: for example, *suzhi gao*, "high quality"; *suzhi di*, "low quality"; and *geren suzhi*, "personal quality" (Griffiths & Zeuthen, 2014); or *xinli suzhi*, "psychological quality"; *sixiang suzhi*, "quality of consciousness"; *suzhi jiao*, "educational quality"; *wenhua suzhi*, "cultural quality"; *guomin suzhi*, "quality of the national population"; and *suzhi fuping*, "suzhi poverty relief" (Hairong, 2003).

The concept of *suzhi* is used across such a wide conceptual range that the term can indicate either neoliberalism or its antithesis (Hairong, 2003). It can be best understood in the context of governance, being reflective of not only authoritarian and neoliberal perspectives but also multiple influential approaches that incorporate Confucian, Legalist, and Daoist thought. These historical features being more evident in non-state realms such as self-management and a commitment to family and other relationships (Kipnis, 2007).

High-quality *suzhi* is strongly linked to educational status and other markers of successful self-development (Kipnis, 2007). However, there are subtle social markers that make it difficult to attain this degree of *suzhi*. As a rule, a high level of income alone cannot move an individual up the *suzhi* hierarchy if people consider that person as lacking the educational, familial, and other status markers that reflect self-cultivation. So, there is no definitive and objective way to assess the quality of *suzhi*: "In most instances, the politics of suzhi evaluation are the politics of arbitrary personal power, administrative fiat, or contested public standards" (p. 392).

Again, this tendency contradicts the goal of creating productive, autonomous, and entrepreneurial citizens, as the current deployment of *suzhi* enforces class divisions. With regard to a technical skill set, it is market demand that determines the features and quality of *suzhi* required of the individual. That is often assessed using material and financial criteria. The individual is not, however, fully autonomous; there are limits across all groups, including that of the elites, in the service of maintaining the hegemony of the Communist Party of China. It would seem that a disproportionate amount of high *suzhi* is found among the Han people and also among selected elites from the minority ethnic groups who adopt Han values.

The politically acceptable form of *suzhi* is also antithetical to the form of neoliberalism that envisions a less activist state yet leaves markets relatively free from arbitrary state intervention (Kipnis, 2007). In that sense, it is consistent with a strand of Chinese culture where the crown lies uneasily on the heads of all who hold power. The psychological cost of *suzhi*, therefore, can be quite high, given the state's selective retreat from the provision of social services and the sense that the average citizen is at the mercy of the market and often lacks the resources to meet its demands. *Suzhi* is also a source of stress for elites given its fluid definition and the risk of its sudden and seemingly capricious devaluation and the concomitant loss of status and power they might experience. Such stressors call for much psychological resilience, the kind of which Chinese have embodied in their concept of *chiku*, "eating bitterness."

One could argue the raison d'etre for the presence of most Africana persons' presence in China is to improve themselves; to enhance their quality of *suzhi*. Allaya is a 32-year-old Malian man with an elementary school education, who runs his own export business. He has lived in China since 2005 with his East African wife and two children. Before coming to China he worked as a trader in Mali and then in other West African countries as an importer of consumer goods.

Allaya speaks to how he has grown as follows:

> I am more experienced about business. I see a lot so I can use my mind to do better. I know more and I think more about what I see with people and how they act, how they do business.

Venus is a 44-year-old African American woman who teaches English. She has extensive experience in theater arts and has lived in China for 1 year. She had a peripatetic upbringing and lived and worked in various cities in the United States. Prior to coming to China, she worked in North Africa and Western Europe as a teacher in international schools.

> I have a sense of pride; did not turn tail and go home. I made friends, I can communicate in Chinese, I can fend for myself. I have always done that but doing that in China is not easy.

Chiku: Eating Bitterness

The term *chiku*, "eating bitterness," speaks to stoic persistence and confidence in the face of severe obstacles to striving to achieve one's life outcomes, and it also speaks to a phlegmatic acceptance of limits on one's aspirations. As one person explains:

> People without pressure will fall away; a well without pressure will not spurt oil. But you must go step-by-step; you must walk on the road in an earnest and down-to-earth manner. I'm this kind of person. I rely on my own perspective and striving; there is nothing I can't do. But only if you are willing to do things in the proper sequence, with perseverance and the right attitude, can you do it. It will never be the case that you get positive feedback every time you invest effort in something; sometimes you will try very hard and not get any results at all. But if you don't try you can be sure that you will never get anything back. Life is fair, we all have 24 hours per day, but how we live is up to us. Life is never easy, never plain sailing. You've just got to strive with all your might. I always say, "There is nothing difficult in front of me. When the car is at the bottom of the mountain, there must surely be a road; you don't need to think too much about it."
>
> (Griffiths & Zeuthen, 2014, pp. 156–157)

At its core, eating bitterness ideally concerns spirit, tradition, and persistence, while avoiding the fleeting temptations of a networked, narcissistic culture in which the only markers of success are material goods and credentials attesting to high levels of cognitively oriented skills. It involves accepting limits and disappointments so there is a stoic component to it. It appears to spurn the material oriented middle-class notion of success, promoting instead inner growth, self-awareness, and the acceptance of limits. This approach is ancient and reflects Taoist and Buddhist themes, as opposed to Confucian or communist values. The latter two, "[frame] individuals only in terms of their roles within social collectives, such as relations to the family, the community, and the nation," according to Griffiths and Zeuthen (2014, p. 153). Furthermore, "success is not about having the best strategy or coming out on top, nor is it about fulfilling one's responsibility to society or self-sacrifice; it is about doing your best, and being in touch with yourself" (p. 153).

This concept has a long history in China, first as a fundamentally rural virtue and later as a legitimizing force behind the CPC, with its imperative for sacrifice in the struggle to establish the People's Republic and through the Cultural Revolution (Hairong, 2003). Urban development came at the cost of rural development, with the understanding that such sacrifices were necessary: "It was used to mobilize China's masses during Mao's rise to power and the Cultural Revolution" (Griffiths & Zeuthen, 2014, p. 145). Bitterness in this context was defined as "the capacity to endure hardship, make sacrifices, and work hard. We argue, however, that bitterness-eating discourse today has new meanings, and increasingly refers to self-development without sacrifice to a higher purpose" (p. 145).

With the ascent of market philosophies under Deng Xiaoping, the state receded somewhat from its longtime role as the dominant arbitrator of the rural–urban divide. Rural society was long seen by the elites as representing a harsh reality (*suzhi di*) in relation to a quality lifestyle (*suzhi gao*) that is removed from physical hardship, which was seen as the defining characteristic of a middle-class lifestyle. This vision was entrenched in the household registration system, which made it difficult to traverse the rural–urban divide and move from the level of *suzhi di* to *suzhi gao* (Griffiths & Zeuthen, 2014).

Despite this decoupling, *suzhi* is selectively deployed to serve the interest of the development of the economy. One can be admired socially for the decision to eat bitterness in the service of personal goals, without necessarily observing how such behaviors serve neoliberal policies at the expense of the long-term interests of individuals (Dilts, 2011). In China, there is beginning to emerge the unwitting replication of Western culture with its emphasis on materialism alongside the marginalization of the emotional.

Given that, one will find Africana persons who have not been successful in China who to some degree manifest elements of eating bitterness. An interesting variant of this was evident among some undocumented Gambian workers who were unsuccessful in China. Omar (Haugen & Diederich, 2016), discusses his experiences in China:

> I didn't hide it from my family, and they told other who asked them about. If anyone ask, I tell them I was in China. I tell them "China is mafan [Chinese for trouble]," Some people ask me about China, and I educate them. China is bad. Business is okay in China, but hustling is bad. . . . Yesterday, people said "You are a coward for going home from China!" people say: "You are afraid." They can ruin your reputation and ruin your life. You come back with stress, and people put more stress upon you. What people think about being in China is that you are sitting around because you are too lazy to find a job. . . . I went to the visa dealer and told him everything about what China is like. He stopped selling visas to China.

In summary, China offers much to the world in terms of its traditions, its seeming commitment to *suzhi*, and its promulgation of a perspective that speaks to the oft-denied necessity of eating bitterness. Its history biases it to be heavily invested in the control of knowledge despite the urgent demands for it to be more creative and the democratizing of knowledge that should flow from such permissiveness. Given the historical record, it struggles with managing the tradeoffs of being open to new ideas and the destabilizing effects that such influx of ideas and practices can engender. Its flirtation with neoliberalism within an authoritarian structure that wishes for creativity but is suspicious and at times indifferent to subjectivities speaks to this dilemma.

While "classical neoliberalism" speaks to the creation of autonomous individuals, such autonomy is interpreted in China in the context of one's relationship to the market. Individual autonomy is limited to the choices an individual makes about material production and consumption. Current state policies allow one to be an entrepreneur of the self in the economic realm but not in the sociopolitical realm (Dilts, 2011). This contrasts with Sen's (1989) capabilities argument that skill development and self-management is ideally in the service of improving an individual's ability to be free.

Here, one is confronted by the many ideological contradictions regarding development in China. Historically, there has always been an interest in improving the quality of the individual as a moral and productive being in the service of embracing modernity for the sake of building a vibrant China, rather than as a good solely for the sake of the individual (Hui, 2009; Mitter, 2004). One consequence of the neoliberal turn, in China and elsewhere, is that it has led to a selective withdrawal of the state that is manifested in less investment in caring for the vulnerable and in the development of human capabilities, functions now subjugated to the needs of the market and the initiative and resourcefulness of individuals in their roles as entrepreneurs of the self.

Thus, each individual is a potential entrepreneur defined increasingly by the quality of his or her productive relationship to the market (Hairong, 2003) and by an understanding that there will be no questioning of the political arrangements. There is little value attached to, or investment in, the subjectivities of the individual outside of market-mediated needs (Dilts, 2011). Such an individual is highly constrained, because his or her individuality is vulnerable given an orientation toward a market culture that features "the incorporation of all subjective potential, the capacity to communicate, to feel, to create, to think, into productive powers for capital" (Read, 2009, p. 33). According to De Genova (2012), who refers to the ideas of Giorgio Agamben: "What remains when human existence, while yet alive, is nonetheless stripped of all the encumbrances of social location and juridical identity, and thus bereft of all the qualifications for properly political inclusion and belonging?" (pp. 132–133).

These policy changes have created a "floating population" composed of millions of rural laborers from China's vast hinterlands who serve as the backbone of the labor force necessary to drive China's economic modernization (Davin, 2009). They are actively encouraged to migrate to urban areas to address a seemingly insatiable demand for low-cost labor and to generate demand for goods and services. In offering their services to the market, they are encouraged to improve the quality of their skills, increase their income, and reap the concomitant material and status benefits (Simpson, 2013; Taylor, 2011).

This stance also applies to Africana persons in China who seek knowledge, treasure, and high levels of *suzhi*, but who must also eat bitterness. China becomes a site for both self-improvement and self-awareness. It is a laboratory where many of the issues they struggled with at home, such as the ethical cost of state support in the context of the disciplinary mandates of neoliberalism, are being re-enacted. Here, the individual has a greater sense of autonomy than at home, and China offers the possibility, if carefully embraced, to contribute to China's attempts to engage the world as a creative and ethical partner.

References

Adams, C. J. (2014). Afro-Caribbean people in China: Away from home and at home with self. *Caribbean Journal of Psychology*, *6*(1), 1–20.

Adams, C. J. (2015). Structure and agency: Africana immigrants in China. *Journal of Pan African Studies*, *7*(10), 85–108.

Ademoyo, A. (2009). The ontological imperative for the new African diaspora. In I. Okpewho & N. Nzegwu (Eds.), *The new African diaspora* (pp. 501–518). Bloomington, IN: Indiana University Press.

Anagnost, A. (2004). The corporeal politics of quality (suzhi). *Public Culture*, *16*(2), 189–208.

Anonymous. (2009a). NetEase interview with Shanghai black girl Lou Jing. Retrieved from www.chinahush.com/2009/09/15/netease-interview-with-shanghai-black-girl-lou-jing/

Anonymous. (2009b). Shanghai black girl Lou Jing. Retrieved from www.chinahush.com/2009/09/01/shanghai-black-girl-lou-jing/

Anonymous. (2013). What is it like to be black and gay in China? Retrieved from www.quora.com/What-is-it-like-to-be-black-and-gay-in-China

Ariga, K., Ohtake, F., Sasaki, M., & Wu, Z. (2012). Wage growth through job hopping in China. Discussion Paper Series, Forschungsinstitut zur Zukunft der Arbeit, No. 7104. Retrieved from http://hdl.handle.net/10419/69464

Baijia, Z. (2009). The evolution of China's diplomacy and foreign relations in the era of reform, 1976–2005. In Y. Hao, G. Wei, & L. Dittmer (Eds.), *Asia in the new millennium: Challenges to Chinese foreign policy: Diplomacy, globalization, and the next world power* (pp. 15–33). Lexington, KY: University Press of Kentucky.

Bakewell, O. (2010). Some reflections on structure and agency in migration theory. *Journal of Ethnic and Migration Studies*, *36*(10), 1689–1708.

Bauman, Z. (1991). *Modernity and ambivalence*. London, UK: Polity Press.

Binkley, S. (2011). Psychological life as enterprise: Social practice and the government of neo-liberal interiority. *History of the Human Sciences*, *24*(3), 83–102.

Bodomo, A. (2012). *Africans in China*. Amherst, NY: Cambria Press.

Castillo, R. (2016). How many Africans are in Guangzhou? Retrieved from https://africansinchina.net/how-many-africans-are-there-in-guangzhou/

Cisse, D. (2015). African traders in Yiwu: Their trade networks and their role in the distribution of "made in China" products in Africa. *Journal of Pan African Studies*, 7(10), 44–64.

Cooke, F., Saini, D., & Wang, J. (2014). Talent management in China and India: A comparison of management perceptions and human resource practices. *Journal of World Business*, *49*(2), 225–235.

Crossley, P. (1990). Thinking about ethnicity in early China. *Late Imperial China*, *11*(1), 1–35.

Davin, D. (2009). Internal migration in China. *DevISSues*, *11*(2), 13–15. Retrieved from https://issuu.com/devissues/docs/devissues_volume_11__number_2__nov_

De Genova, N. (2012). Bare life, labor-power, mobility, and global space: Toward a Marxian anthropology? *CR: The New Centennial Review*, *12*(3), 129–152.

de Haas, H. (2014). Migration theory: Quo vadis? (DEMIG project paper 24, University of Oxford: International Migration Institute).

Dikotter, F. (1992). *The discourse of race in modern China*. London, UK: Hurst & Company.

Dilts, A. (2011). From "entrepreneur of the self" to "care of the self": Neo-liberal governmentality and Foucault's ethics. *Foucault Studies*, *12*, 130–146.

Echeruo, M. (1999). An African diaspora: The ontological project. In I. Okpewho, C. Davies, & A. Mazrui (Eds.), *The African diaspora* (pp. 3–18). Bloomington, IN: Indiana University Press.

Fallows, J. (2016). China's great leap backward. Retrieved from www.theatlantic.com/magazine/archive/2016/12/chinas-great-leap-backward/505817/

Fennell, V. (2013). Race: China's question and problem. *Review of Black Political Economy*, *40*, 245–275.

Foster, R. (2016). The catastrophe of neo-liberalism: Finance, emancipation and disintegration. *Philosophy and Social Criticism*, *43*(2), 123–143.

Freire, P. (2000). *Pedagogy of the oppressed*. New York, NY: Continuum.

Griffiths, M., & Zeuthen, J. (2014). Bitter sweet China: New discourses of hardship and social organization. *Journal of Current Chinese Affairs*, *43*(4), 143–174.

Haimei, S. (2011). Inflow of international immigrants challenges China's immigration policy. Retrieved from www.brookings.edu/research/opinions/2011/09/08-china-immigrants-shen

Hairong, Y. (2003). Neoliberal governmentality and neohumanism: Organizing suzhi/value flow through labor recruitment networks. *Cultural Anthropology*, *18*(4), 493–523.

Hall, S. (1990). Cultural identity and diaspora. In J. Rutherford (Ed.), *Identity, community, culture and difference* (pp. 222–237). London, UK: Lawrence & Wishart.

Haugen, H. (2015). Destination China: The country adjusts to its new migration reality. Retrieved from http://migrationpolicy.org/article/destination-china-country-adjusts-its-new-migration-reality

Haugen, H., & Diederich, M. (2016). Returning home. Retrieved from https://uturnasia.com/2016/01/22/returning-home/

Hevi, E. (1962). *An African student in China*. New York, NY: Frederick Praeger Publishers.

Hui, W. (2009). *The end of the revolution: China and the limits of modernity*. London, UK: Verso.

Jayasuriya, S. (2006). Identifying Africans in Asia: What's in a name? *African and Asian Studies*, *5*(3/4), 275–303.

Kim, N. (2009). Multicultural challenges in Korea: The current stage and a prospect. *International Migration*, *52*(2), 100–121.

Kipnis, A. (2007). Neoliberalism reified: Suzhi discourse and tropes of neoliberalism in the People's Republic of China. *Journal of the Royal Anthropological Institute*, *13*, 383–400.

Kleinman, A., Yan, Y., Jun, J., Lee, S., Zhang, E., Tianshu, P., . . . Jinhau, G. (Eds.). (2011). *Deep China: The moral life of the person: What anthropology and psychiatry tell us about China today*. Berkeley, CA: University of California Press.

Mitter, R. (2004). *A bitter revolution: China's struggle with the modern world*. Oxford, UK: Oxford University Press.

Morais, I. (2009). Chinese "Wahala": The tribulations of Nigerian "Bushfallers" in a Chinese territory. *Journal of Global Cultural Studies*, *5*, 2–22.

Myers, S., Jr., Xiaoyan, G., & Cruz, B. (2013). Ethnic minorities, race, and inequality in China: A new perspective on racial dynamics. *Review of Black Political Economy*, *40*, 231–244.

Phan, P., Zhou, J., & Abrahamson, E. (2010). Creativity, innovation and entrepreneurship in China. *Management and Organizational Review*, *62*(2), 175–194.

Read J. (2009). A genealogy of homo-economicus: Neoliberalism and the production of subjectivity. *Foucault Studies*, *6*, 25–36.

Sen, A. (1989). Development as capability expansion. *Journal of Development Planning*, *19*, 41–58.

Sewell, W., Jr. (1992). A theory of structure: Duality, agency, and transformation. *American Journal of Sociology*, *98*(1), 1–29.

Simon, D., & Cao, C. (2009). China's future: Have talent, will thrive. *Issues in Science and Technology*. Retrieved from http://issues.org/26-1/simon/

Simpson, N. (2013). Happiness and migration. In A. Constant & K. Zimmerman (Eds.), *International handbook on the economics of migration* (pp. 393–407). Northampton, MA: Edward Elgar Publishing.

Spence, J. (1984). Spence on Needham. *Isis*, *75*(1), 171–189.

Spence, J. (1990). *The search for modern China*. New York, NY: W.W. Norton & Company.

Suttmeier, R., Cao, C., & Simon, D. (2006, April 7). Knowledge Innovation and the Chinese academy of sciences. *Science*, *312*, 58–59. Retrieved from www.sciencemag.org/cgi/content/full/312/5770/58

Taylor, G. (2011). Migration studies unit working papers: China's floating migrants: Updates from the 2005 1% Population Sample Survey. Retrieved from www.lse.ac.uk/government/research/resgroups/MSU/documents/workingPapers/WP_2011_07.pdf

Wang, D. (2011). The dilemma of time: Student-centered teaching in the rural classroom in China. *Teaching and Teacher Education*, *27*(1), 157–164.

Wang, F. (2010). China's population destiny: The looming crisis. *Current History*, *109*(728), 244–251.

Wang, H. (2011). China's new talent strategy: Impact on China's development and its global exchanges. *SAIS Review*, *31*, 49–64.

Washington, S. (2009). A new kind of idol Lou Jing. Retrieved from http://parlourmagazine.com/2009/09/a-new-kind-of-idol-lou-jing/

Wyatt, D. (2009). *The Blacks of premodern China*. Philadelphia, PA: University of Philadelphia Press.

Wyatt, D. (2012). The past, present, and future Blacks of China. Retrieved from https://africansinchina.net/2016/07/12/talk-don-wyatt-the-past-present-and-future-blacks-of-china/

Yao, S. (2000). Economic development and poverty reduction in China over 20 years of reforms. *Economic Development and Cultural Change*, *48*(3), 447–474.

Yongyu, H. (1973). Owl. Retrieved from www.wikiart.org/en/huang-yongyu/owl-1973

Yuan, H. (2008). Chinese ethnicities and their culture: An overview. DLPS Publications. Paper 23. Retrieved from http://digitalcommons.wku.edu/dlps_fac_pub/23/

Zang, X. (2015). *Ethnicity in China: A critical introduction*. Malden, MA: Polity Press.

Zhou, R. (2009). Seeing red over black angel. Retrieved from www.chinadaily.com.cn/opinion/2009-09/18/content_8711576.htm

6 Contemporary Blackness in China

Psychosocial Perspectives, Aspirations, and Constraints

China is experiencing a demand for creative and innovative workers as its economy shifts from low-end manufacturing to generating high-end goods and services. A host of Africana workers, among others, are responding to this demand in areas such as technological services, product development, management training, English language instruction, and exporting goods among other fields. In doing this work, they derive a level of satisfaction, knowledge, and material wealth not possible in their home countries. They must however effectively manage China's wariness toward the foreigner and its default racism. Managing the opportunities and limits gives rise to ambivalence that must be effectively managed if the Africana worker is to succeed in China.

China is often perceived as stressing its cultural homogeneity and perceiving itself as being superior to the West and to non-Chinese peoples. Foreigners in general were viewed either disparagingly or with ambivalence, and hierarchies of peoples were established, with Black, meaning dark-skinned, persons being viewed disdainfully as being primitive (Dikotter, 1992). Whites from the West were historically viewed with ambivalence, looked down on as foreigners but admired for their scientific and technical prowess (Dikotter, 1992; Fennell, 2013). This ambivalence is also informed by China's history of struggle against the West, and its identification with developing countries, many with Africana populations that have also experienced the traumatic effects of Western imperialism (Gallicchio, 2000). The influx of foreigners including Africana workers is a challenge to China's ambivalence to cultural difference.

Contemporary Africana Population in China: Definition

Bodomo (2012), in his pioneering work on Africans in China, notes that defining Africana persons in the Chinese context is quite challenging. Many Chinese people have a tendency to define all dark-skinned persons as African regardless of their country of origin. Bodomo (2010) provides an expansive definition:

> [T]he term African as it is used here is first and foremost meant to refer to someone who is a citizen of any of the countries in Africa. It also includes people who are not citizens of any of the countries in Africa but who consider themselves to be from Africa or to be of African origin.
>
> (p. 4)

I prefer to limit the term *African* to persons born in continental Africa and use the term *Africana* to include them and anyone claiming Africana heritage but not born in Africa. This would include members of the vast and diverse African diaspora.

Africana networks, especially those in southern China are organized around a multiplicity of identifications including nation, region, race/ethnicity, and religion. This multiplicity of potential identity claims allows Africana migrants in China to construct and tactically deploy a hierarchy of identity postures in a given locale to advance their respective self-projects (Bodomo, 2012; Torres-Saillant, 2009). For example, Afro-Caribbean migrants in China may think of themselves as persons of Africana heritage from a particular country or region, or as New World Blacks or simply as Black.

Size of Africana Population in China

It is difficult to get an accurate sense of the size of the Africana community in China as no official statistics are available, but unofficial estimates place the population at more than 20,000 persons (Skeldon, 2012; Wang, 2010). This is in the context of an official statistic of 600,000 foreigners residing in China, according to the 2010 census (Haugen, 2015). Castillo (2016) notes that there does not appear to be any centralized government source that can provide a reliable statistic regarding the size of the large Africana community in Guangzhou.

Composition of Africana Population

The Africana population is distributed mainly on the east coast of China, with the largest community, consisting mostly of traders, residing in Guangzhou and its environs. Castillo (2016), notes that this southern China cohort is made up of three broad groupings of Africana businesspersons. The first has been in China for an extended period of time, usually over 3 years. There is another subgroup, which is the largest, consisting of transient persons many of whom are exporters shuttling between West African countries and southern China. The third subgroup consists of what he refers to as "first timers" and "over stayers"; the latter group consisting of individuals whose visas has expired and who are now considered to be staying illegally in China. Complicating attempts to count Africana persons via country of origin is the fact many persons of Africana heritage have entered China on passports that would not allow one to immediately classify them as Africana persons.

The population of traders is predominantly African, unmarried young males, with Nigerians comprising the largest national group (Bodomo, 2012). The trader population is quite diverse in terms of religion, ethnicity, education, and migratory patterns. Some traders engage in shuttle migration, moving back and forth between home and China, while others are full-time residents and have Chinese wives and children born in China (Adams, 2015).

There is also a relatively small, culturally diverse, and physically dispersed Africana network of mostly corporate business professionals in Shanghai (Adams, 2015). They maintain electronic links among themselves and there is a vibrant organization that serves them an information exchange and that organizes social events and community assistance projects in the Shanghai area. These well-paid technocrats are predominantly single professionals from Africa and the diaspora; many are trained in Western educational institutions. Their creative and technical skills are in high demand by Western and Chinese corporations, universities, and private schools in areas such as information technology, design, sales, financial services, and foreign language skills. Most are on relatively short-term assignments, while a small cohort have been in China for many years. These mostly formally employed technocrats have the legal right to work in China, but like the overwhelming majority of foreigners in China, they have short-term visas that must be renewed annually.

Africana teachers of English, like Africana students, can be found across China. West Africans, specifically Nigerians, dominate in Guangzhou in Guangdong Province, and significant numbers of North Africans and increasingly West Africans are found in Yiwu in Zhejiang Province. There are smaller groups of Africans dispersed within Shanghai and, to a lesser degree, Beijing.

There is also the longest standing community of Africana persons in China residing in Macau, that has been in existence since the seventeenth century, with most of its members being from Lusophone countries, but with a relatively recent influx of Nigerians (Morais, 2009; Pinheiro & Chaplin, 2015). The history of this small community is quite instructive in terms of the Africana presence in China. Portugal, a European pioneer in the enslavement of Africans, established a colony in Macau with both African and Chinese enslaved persons. The Africans were also employed as soldiers and as sailors working on Portuguese sailing vessels (Morais, 2009). Many were used as marine soldiers in Portuguese battles on behalf of some Japanese elements in their internal wars (Pinheiro & Chaplin, 2015).

Macau over the centuries developed and maintained a substantive trade relationship with Portugal and with its former African colonies, resulting in many from these countries residing in Macau. A subgroup consisting of civil servants stayed on after the departure of the Portuguese and has the right to reside permanently in Macau. Africana persons, including those in Macau, have been experienced ambivalently by the Chinese across time, with doubts about how civilized they were and concerns about them marrying the Chinese (Morais, 2009). This sat alongside a sense of their contributions to Macau in the context of a long history of inter-ethnic interactions, in contrast to the lack of such sustained exposure on the part of people from the Chinese mainland. As a consequence, there is a positive bias toward Africana persons in Macau, but it is seemingly restricted to those from Lusophone countries (Morais, 2009). Nigerian students who have arrived in Macau relatively recently have experienced difficulty in obtaining work upon graduating, given a negative perception of them by the Macanese (Morais, 2009).

This influx speaks to the worldwide growth of individuals traveling abroad for economic, intellectual, and other forms of self-development. Such aspiration-driven movements are evident among Africana persons in China. Also evident is the psychological costliness of the pursuit of their aspirations.

Aspirations and Their Purpose

Individuals aspire, however modestly, to realize the dream they have for themselves, their loved ones, and their communities. These aspirations are in part a product of imagination and cultural context, and inform the decision of a given individual, and that of millions of others, to leave the limiting and frustrating certainties of home. Psychological, social, and material resources are used to facilitate the pursuit of enhanced capabilities that will grant individuals the substantive agency needed to realize their long-thwarted aspirations.

Complexity of Aspirations

Collinson (in Castles, 2010) notes the complexity of the aspirational process:

> the inter-linkages between different migration streams: the importance of agency, autonomy, perceptions, cultural and historical factors and institutional constraints; the complex multi-level and transitional level of migration; and the importance of social groups and relationship-including migration networks-for shaping migration dynamics and migration experiences, straddling migration, "sending," "receiving," and "transit" locations, and a range of actors within them.
>
> (p. 1573)

Africana persons in China are there for reasons that include but are not limited to the pursuit of material gain. Harry, a 26-year-old French entrepreneur with West African heritage, spoke to his aspiration to be autonomous as motivating him to leave France for China:

> France does not evolve much so I know why I left. I was looking for opportunities for young people. I was happy, very happy to leave. The very first time I could make something happen to myself; create something in China without parental help.

Raoul is a 35-year-old Guadeloupian man with a postgraduate degree in the arts, and he has lived and worked in China for the past 5 years as an art director in various media related and design jobs. He stressed the need for self-development and artistic expression:

> (I am) always thinking that I am different. I am eager; starving to do different. (I) must have something artistic to do.

Factors That Facilitate the Realization of Aspirations

The capacity to enact a given aspiration is also contingent on features of the individual's psychological repertoire alongside the contribution of social and economic factors. Following is a discussion of six psychological factors that contribute to the framing and pursuit of aspirations.

The Dream

The first of these is the dream, the idea for the self that goes beyond the acquisition of the technical capabilities that facilitate the attaining of economic goals (de Haas, 2014). Diverse cultural images and narratives about the foreign that gush from the globalized multimedia hydrant inform such a dream, that is in turn authenticated by the narratives of those who left and have done well (or not so well). Here is how Garba, a 35-year-old Nigerien administrator, explained the impetus to leave:

> I grew up in a culture (Niger) where going abroad is the ultimate goal. That is an incredible achievement; equated with being a success, people speak highly of it. Going to Nigeria was an important goal; getting a scholarship; going abroad. The motivation was to just go abroad to a foreign country; no particular agenda.

So, while the constraints in terms of capabilities and resources are real, it is often the accentuated lack, heightened by the globalized images of possibilities, that feeds the aspirations resulting in migrating. The dream can speak to a not necessarily conscious need, to broaden the experience of belong in ways not possible at home. This was evident among some Nigerians in southern China who, having achieved economic stability, had keenly felt aspirations to become substantive members of the Chinese community, in addition to their ties to their ethnic, national, and Africana communities in China. Aspirations therefore continue to evolve and to become more differentiated over time. This speaks in part to the developmentally driven growth of the individual.

Developmental Imperatives

Developmental imperatives inform the nature and quality of the dream that drives the individual's aspirations.

Urgency of Youth

For the young adult, there is urgency to the need to explore a range of possibilities in the process of self-definition and development. This might very well include the age-typical bias of leaping before looking, as was evident with John, the Nigerian, who came to China knowing no one and lacking a job or place to say, but was unperturbed by this leap into the relatively unknown. He managed to acquire a job and a residence with 12 hours of arriving in Guangzhou. A Ugandan teacher of English, also using the pseudonym John, with an abundance of self-confidence and curiosity, went sight unseen to teach in a community in central China that had apparently never had actual contact with an Africana person:

> I got a teaching job in northern China. They had a band to welcome me, there was a red carpet. If they really like you, they can do really nice things for you. I got a nice apartment and they bought me clothes. I got the same reception at a second school. I have tried to understand Chinese culture and they sense that I understand how we are different and that I understand their expectations.

The experiences of John, as a teacher illustrate the interaction of personal qualities with socioeconomic factors. He is socially adept, technically skilled, and resilient, allowing him to take advantage of opportunities and also to accept the need for compromise when necessary. Such self-skills and vulnerabilities are long in the making and preceded the Africana individual's arrival in China.

Cumulative Effect of Development

Individuals' histories of development impact on their ability to adaptively manage the conflicts inherent in being away from home. Where such individuals have been embedded in family and social relationships that have contributed to them developing adaptive strategies for managing loss in the pursuit of self-growth, they tend to be quite resilient. So, Renee is a 32-tyear-old African American woman with a postgraduate degree in education, and she has worked as a teacher. Working in China for the past 2 years, initially as a teacher of English, Renee now works as a curricula development and training manager and is required to travel extensively in East Asia. She made the following observation:

> I did not see myself repeating the mistakes of my mother—premature pregnancy. My grandparents were a big influence in breaking that cycle. I went to Catholic school until eighth grade, not to public school with poor peers. I thought Good Riddance when I left the United States. I did not like how the media portrayed Black culture, and I wanted to experience a difference culture. I felt sad that I was leaving my younger sister, felt I was letting her down but it was something for her to look up to.
>
> Renee

Given that most of the individuals I spoke to were under the age of 35 and were university graduates, they are probably biased to make audacious moves and are not overly preoccupied with concerns around failure or melancholia. At the same time, long-standing unresolved conflicts between a wish to be audacious that is in tension with a history of conservative socialization will continue to influence and possibly limit chance-taking behavior. Given that many of these individuals come from cultures with a history of migration, it is not clear as to how they are socialized to deal with the challenges that they too will face as migrants.

So, developmental considerations inform aspirations throughout the life cycle, and this is evident with Perline, a 41-year-old teacher from the Caribbean, who took stock of her life and felt a sense of underachievement. While she was professionally well respected in her home country, money was a challenge, and she felt unfulfilled and lacking in self-revelatory challenges: "My country is not growing. Financially it is not feasible. I was happy I left." She was encouraged by her sister to leave so that she could explore the possibility of having an enriched life. Perline did much research among members of her global-spanning network and made the carefully considered decision to move to China to teach, learn Chinese, and start a business venture with a friend already established there. Here, one observes the more reflective and considered approach to life that is developmentally appropriate for an adult approaching middle age that does not however, rule out a break with the past.

Character Styles

A third factor is the influence of character style on the breadth of the aspirations imagined and the capacity to adaptively manage the ambivalences generated. There is an irreducible level of melancholy experienced in leaving home, no matter how inspiring the motivations to do so (Beltsiou, 2016). Much of what is familiar will be relinquished, but this sits alongside an excitement about the possibilities for self-development in the uncertainties that the individual is going to warily embrace.

Natasha, a 31-year-old teacher of Jamaican and American heritage, spoke of her need to be distinct as a motivating factor: "China was the place to me. I wanted a language that would help me in the long run; something that would set me apart from anyone else." Such an individual has an emotional economy well fueled with curiosity and resiliency and will strive to adaptively manage the vicissitudes of the pursuit.

Bill, a 39-year-old African American, reported that he came to China to escape the limits of a racist Los Angeles, and with much pain, he left children and a steady if unfulfilling career in construction. He makes a somewhat precarious living as an informal teacher of English, but exults in his sense of freedom and the possibilities of seeing the world from a less racist perspective, compared to Los Angeles. Bill feels that he is respected as an American in Shanghai and that he can make an honest living, grow intellectually, and in addition have a culturally diverse set of friends. In both cases here, one observes a character style with an orientation toward difference, a curiosity about the unfamiliar, and an interest in developing new relationships (Grinberg & Grinberg, 1982).

Capabilities

In addition to a particular mind-set, adequate capabilities are crucial for the individual to realize aspirations of being a successful migrant or foreign worker. In Sen's (1989) formulations, to be successful in life, the individual must have the necessary capabilities that are the basis of the robust sense of agency that facilitates being free and experiencing good-enough well-being. Many Africana persons in China are able to develop and deploy the capabilities necessary to acquire knowledge and reasonable wealth but also to be socially confident and adept. So, in addition to earning academic degrees and money, many subjects spoke to the development of social and psychological skills.

Cibana, a 45-year-old banking consultant from central Africa noted, "I have a much more complex way of seeing the world. I am more open to new ideas and I am better at knowing what to hold on to and when to compromise." Such capabilities are, however, often predicated on having developed a solid foundation of the desired socio-emotional, critical thinking, and adaptive skills, prior to coming to China. They inform the evolution and successful pursuit of aspirations once living in China. Many of the subjects attained a college degree prior to coming to China; some had considerable work and travel experience prior to arriving. The experiences of Venus, a 44-year-old African American teacher and artist, are illustrative and fairly typical. She had attained her degree and worked in various regions of the United States; she then moved to North Africa, where she taught in an international school prior to coming to China. Given such experiences their sojourn in China tended to be enhanced by the capabilities they had prior to arriving there.

A lack of capabilities in some aspect of cognitive or socio-emotional functioning often foretold unfulfilling experiences in China. So, traders with poor commercial skills and lacking the savvy to access high-quality support networks tended to be unsuccessful in China. I also observed the pattern of Africana persons struggling despite being intellectually well prepared upon arriving in China and doing well at school or in the technical job market. Such individuals brought with them unresolved conflicts around relating and chance taking in the social sphere and continued to struggle in this regard.

Another type of impediment is that of lacking the technical skills that are in demand exacerbated by the individual not making attempts to acquire those skills in China. Such individuals are evident in the Africana community in southern China, who failed at trading or dropped out of school. They live precarious lives, often no better than their experiences in their respective home countries. One could therefore speculate that individuals like Bill, mentioned above, with limited technical capabilities and a lack of formal credentialing, would probably not do well in China in the medium-to-long run.

Status and Class

Status and class standing are crucial facilitators of the shaping and actualizing of aspirations; both are linked to mobility, access, and income. The attaining of a desirable status level can be aspirational and therefore motivates the individual to commit to a particular course of work. In some cases, it is the outcome of the work rather than the work itself that can garner the type of status sought. John, the Ugandan who teaches English, is in a position that does not carry particularly a high status in China; he is, however, held in high esteem in his home country due to his ability to purchase and build a family home there with the surplus income earned in China. Equally important for John was his ability to engage high status Chinese individuals who assisted him in improving his earning capacity and in smoothing out visa difficulties. The combination of his character style and his leveraging of his social status enables John to achieve his economic goals in China and enhance his social status in Uganda.

With others, status, although less tied to the social, is equally important, and this was evident among many of the technocrats in Shanghai who were proud of their increased capacity to manage the social demands of being in China. They perceived themselves to be affluent, mobile, and competent compared to when they left their home countries. Cecilia and Wei Wei, two successful Africana women, embody earned status. With these subjects, status was not tightly linked to feedback from Chinese or home country family and friends, although there was that. What mattered most to them was that on reflection, they perceived themselves as attaining a higher status as mature and thoughtful persons than they would have had they not come to China. Here, status is linked to both psychological and social achievements.

For some Africana persons, class is crucial in shaping and achieving aspirations that will convey high status. An important facilitating factor is a long history, beginning at home of being embedded in well-resourced and data-rich networks that will inform the aspirations they own and the means to pursue them. Such networks include family members and others throughout the Africana diaspora, who ensured they were well equipped to handle the vicissitudes of being in China.

Marie, a 31-year-old African American entrepreneur, came from a family that had the resources to travel extensively, including bringing her to China as a young adult. Care was also taken to ensure that she developed an appreciation for cultural diversity, while at the same time ensuring she was proud of being African American. Her family's social and financial capital ensured that she was well positioned to be perceptive, autonomous, and mobile:

> I knew that I wanted to leave California; that I wanted to travel. I wanted to learn Spanish and Chinese. My brother went abroad, so I wanted to do that too. My parents took me to China in 2007. My mom pushed me. I visited Costa Rica. I spoke with a mentor and she told me to go [to China]; including everybody (else) in my support system.

Many subjects who came from such well-endowed networks, such as the Africana technocrats in Shanghai or the successful traders in Guangzhou and Yiwu, would focus on self-development including and beyond the skills needed to acquire financial and technical resources. This was evident in traders and technocrats deeply involved in community work, where one observes an inclination to work across class boundaries both within the Africana community and in outreach and assistance to low-income Chinese persons. Many also reported that despite being worldly, having traveled extensively prior to coming to China, their experiences in China tempered their hereto unacknowledged tendencies to view the world from a privileged Euro American perspective and to be intolerant of other ways of being in the world. These psychosocial developments in turn enabled them to have more diverse and substantive relations, and many sensed that they were viewed more positively and with higher status than peers who had not done such reflective and cross-cultural work.

Relationships

Aspirations therefore cannot be limited to cognitive skills, wealth, and status. So, there exists a subgroup of financially and professionally successful Africana workers who struggle with loneliness given their limited ability to develop substantive and healthy interdependent relationships. To the extent that they are reflective, some will acknowledge that this was a challenge prior to leaving home and that they have re-created the conditions in China that make it difficult to work on the problem. Interacting with this self-imposed limitation is often a failure to learn Chinese, which limits the possibilities for developing a diverse base of healthy relationships. This issue is illustrated in the case of Krystal, a 29-year-old Caribbean science lecturer at a university close to Shanghai. Her upbringing was quite mixed with a focus on intellectual achievement but at the same time it was emotionally quite impoverished:

> As a child I spent a lot of time by myself, and I guess I was closest to my teachers. It has been hard for me to make and keep friends. I have done well intellectually in China; I have achieved what I set out to do here. I keep to myself and hardly socialize, so in that sense not much has changed since leaving home.

Others have more broad-based and mutually gratifying relationships as exemplified by Wei Wei, who has cultivated a diverse and nurturing group of friends that includes native monolingual Chinese speakers. These relations enhanced their status even as they did the same for like-minded peers. Such individuals convey a sense of having either discovered or cultivated aspects of the self that with work enabled them to achieve more and to be resilient in the face of the limitations they experienced in China. This broad-based sense of the self as competent was a crucial self-perception for managing in an adaptive manner the ambivalence they felt about being in China.

Less dramatic is the fate of certain members of the Africana population in China whose economic aspirations have been satisfied, but they are thwarted in their efforts to build healthy interdependent relationships with both Chinese and Africana peers. As a result, they struggle to understand why the experience a sense of not quite being at home wherever they are. Jay, a banker from the Congo, makes the dystopian observation that even if he lived in China for 50 years, he would still be related to as a foreigner. For Africana workers like him, there is a keenly felt sense that wherever they call home has substantial constraints on satisfying their need to belong.

Home: Foundational Legacies as the Root of Ambivalence

Home is a complex construction, as it is an emotionally infused psychic phenomenon that contains passionate attachments to people, places, and ways of being. Those attachments are invariably in some degree of tension with an unblinking sense of home's shortcomings and costs. Regardless of how individuals subjectively understand home, it is an essential component of how they understand themselves and their place in the world. It is a psychological, social, and physical place that is a site of both pleasure and frustration, and it inevitably engenders some degree of ambivalence in the individual. This occurs as that which makes home attractive, such as inclusion, familiarity, and predictability, can also be a source of frustration, given the relative lack of difference and its limited capacity to surprise.

Pleasures of Home

Home offers advantages that support healthy psychological functioning when the individual ventures abroad. It is a place that ideally nurtures and provides a degree of recognition and positive exceptionalism that are predicated on a generous acceptance of the individual. It is capable of tolerating a high degree of irrationality and emotional intensity that would not be accommodated in any other setting, so it is ideally the last refuge for the fantastical and for the acceptance of vulnerability. Perhaps most importantly, it satisfies those human needs to belong and to be recognized, which are fundamental building blocks for a sense of identity.

Kristina, a 46-year-old African American woman, has lived all over the world in her professional role as an international banker and now consultant. She relishes the experience of cultural difference and yet feels it's important to think of herself as being from Brooklyn, New York:

> I have had a global lifestyle for the past twenty years. I need roots to come back to keep me grounded. I will always be a Brooklyn girl wherever I am.

For many, home is psychologically important as it represents continuity and links to a history, however bittersweet it might be. There is a familiar if not always comforting sense of belonging to a psychosocial phenomenon that is larger than the self, and that contributes to a sense of both commonalities and difference. It is a psychosocial space that the individual is attached through relationships and memories. In addition to human relationships, there are also relationships with the environment, including but not limited to food, aesthetics, climate, popular culture, ideology, and administrative systems.

Raoul, from Guadeloupe, finds his country physically enchanting:

> The forest, the ital (vegetarian and organic) food, the rain drops. … I love the rain, the light, the heat of the rain drops.

This, it has been noted, can be the basis of a powerful nostalgia and possible melancholy (Grinberg & Grinberg, 1982). For that to occur home must be unattainable, but for many Africana persons, that is not the case. Raoul's sense of nostalgia lacked a certain potency given that he visits home on a regular basis and noted that after a short sojourn, he was eager to leave.

Home as Constraint

Home implies a set of relationships with an intense emotional valence, some of which are sources of gratification and nurturance, and others of which result in limitation and frustration. It can be, therefore, psychologically costly, given the limits it can place on individual development. First, there are the inevitable constraints that are a feature of group life. For better and sometimes for worse, the individual faces obstacles in the pursuit of love, knowledge, and agency. The price of home, from which many have fled, can be variants of a suffocating and at times austere love and a sparse and equally constrained access to intellectual capital.

King, from central Africa, has bittersweet perceptions of home given his love of his family alongside his exasperation at their unremitting emotional and material demands. As a consequence, he very rarely goes home. One subject, who spoke on condition that she not be identified, is still clearly struggling with the emotional legacy of having been raised by a mentally ill parent in the Caribbean. Other subjects, like Renee, the 32-year-old African American corporate trainer, were glad to have left her home in Detroit with its structural shortcomings:

> It was a challenge to finish high school. … Detroit is the most dangerous city in the United States. There is no comprehension of talking things out.

Mutable Notions of Home

For some, there is a somewhat flexible and multifaceted idea of home that is an outcome of growing up in communities with a multigenerational history of migration. There is, in many cultures, including places such as West Africa, the Americas, and the Caribbean, a discourse around migration that shapes identity in powerful ways. So the idea of, say, Jamaican-ness serves as an important signifier not only for Jamaicans, but also for their offspring living in the Jamaican diaspora. I have many American undergraduate students whose parents are Jamaican who were born and socialized in the United States but define and think of themselves as Jamaican. Many have never visited Jamaica and have no intent of living there permanently. They still however define their identities in relation to Jamaica, while being quite cognizant of the material and citizenship advantages of being American. This cultural sense of self is also illustrated by a Nigerian executive in China who has not lived in his homeland for over 30 years and has no desire to return there permanently but holds fiercely to his sense of being a Nigerian: "It has made me who I am, and I am proud of my roots there."

One can also see that in such cultures, there are potent, long-standing discourses and facilitating structures around dis-embedding and re-embedding in pursuit of the development of a particular aspect of identity. These moves have a pragmatic aspect to them often driven by the pursuit of better living conditions. Stuart Hall (1990) speaks to how these discourses about the self, support both continuity and a refashioning of the self.

> It stands for the endless ways in which Caribbean people have been destined to migrate; it is the signifier of migration itself-of travelling, voyaging and return as fate, as destiny; as the Antillean as the prototype of the modern or postmodern nomad, continually moving between center and periphery.
>
> (Hall, p. 234)

Hierarchy of Attachments to Home

The quality and tenor of the attachments to these diverse aspects of home vary and are hierarchically arranged. The attachment to the idea of a homeland, for instance, might be more gratifying and less conflictual than the attachment to home in terms of family relationships. Or, as is quite common, the attachment to family may be positive and intense, while there is much conflict with the ideology and attendant administrative practices of the state that may result in migration.

Cecilia is a 33-year-old Ugandan college graduate in literature who works in financial services. She has been living in China continuously for the past 5 years and a previous period for 3 years. Before her current stint in China, she resided and worked in southern Africa and India in various management positions. She is married and has two children and made a distinction regarding attachment to family as against country:

> In Uganda, there are no opportunities. I wanted to stay, but the corruption means that even if you were better qualified you could not

> get work. You might never develop, you become a problem, you can't support yourself, others have to support you. I did not want to leave. It was very scary to make the first step to go to South Africa. I thought, if worse comes to worse I will return. I always had a return ticket. If others can go then what about me? We were in our 20s, we lived with our families, everyone is there. (Re going), My mother said no but my father was supportive … he knew my thinking and said I would be ok.

Home, therefore is the midwife of ambivalence, speaking both to comforting familiarity and the unease of stasis.

Ambivalence Regarding Home

Ambivalence is not purely a function of migration, of course, but is engendered by the less-than-fulfilling experiences of home. Longings, conflicts, and dissatisfactions may coexist in the various relationships with home, with no ease of resolution. This sense of ambivalence with regard to home is animated and often refueled—especially by many Africana persons abroad, by way of frequent contact with home using social media. The Africana person in China must manage a paradox increasingly familiar to all who leave the home country in search of increased agency and self-development. The individual realizes that home is loved and must be, to some degree, rejected if one is to live a fulfilling life.

Melinda is a 40-year-old educator of Caribbean American heritage who has lived a very peripatetic lifestyle, working in a given country for an extended period of time and then moving on to the next. She has lived and worked in northern Africa and Southeast Asia and now lives and works in China. Home, from the perspective of family, is a source of much ambivalence for her, as while she is close with some family members, she appears to be in conflict with others. As a consequence, she maintains a distance from home, rarely visiting but communicating frequently with select family members. Also feeding the paradox is the possibility for many that they are able to return home, that in some ineffable way it will always be there, and yet at the same time they are reluctant to return given the awareness of why they left in the first place.

Jocelyn, a 43-year-old Togolese businessman, spoke to his ambivalence when he noted:

> When I was at home you did not have to spend a lot of money to be happy. Now I have to take care of my brothers. I am afraid to go back. There is no good news when I go back, just a lot of problems and I can't fix them all. I went to China to work hard. You do not

> get anything easy. They do not understand or they do not want to understand. Some [relatives] will invoke the spirits against you. Others might try to poison you.

In relation to home, Echeruo (1999) notes:

> The power of the idea lies in the principle of it: that a return is possible forever, whenever, if ever. It is this possibility—this inalienable right to wish to return, to reclaim connections to a lineage, however fractured, that makes one individual a part of a diffuse and disparate collection of persons we call a diaspora.
>
> (p. 14)

This intrapsychic idea reflects the ambivalence of both home as pleasure and caution. It is part of the emotional legacy that accompanies the individual to China.

Home in China

The Need for a Sense of Home

No matter how transient a stay for the foreigner, wherever he or she is located both possesses and lacks homelike attributes. To some degree, foreigners are integrated into a form of community in which they are able to create a sense of home, no matter how precarious it may be. This can be thought of as a state of mind based on social relationships rather than a fixed place (Castillo, 2015).

Once, when traveling to Shanghai, I was requested to bring Black hair products given their unavailability in China. Over time, Mikhaila, who made the request, established the first hair salon in Shanghai that catered to the hair grooming needs of Black women, an important signifier of self and home. Foreigners, such as Africana persons, living in China are almost never permanent residents, with the sense of being legally embraced, but neither are all of them transient.

A foreign worker is not necessarily a migrant, as they are often seen as a threat to notions of a particular exclusive and excluding cultural definition of nationhood (Raijman, 2012). In this regard, the Chinese authorities do not easily facilitate the possibility of foreign workers becoming migrants with the possibility of legal permanency. There is concern that migrants constitute a cultural threat, that they will challenge China's emphasis on cultural harmony and homogeneity, and thus Chinese officials discourage the idea, that for the foreigner, China can become home. The foreigner, however, must establish some spaces with homelike qualities as Mikhaila has done with her salon, and as Emma, the Nigerian community leader, has done in Guangzhou.

Diaspora or Enclave?

The idea of diaspora is a complex and multifaceted container for differences within commonalities and commonalities within difference peculiar to a community of foreigners embedded in a host country (Akyeapong, 2000; Edwards, 2005). It would be premature to claim that the Africana networks in southern China and Shanghai constitute a diaspora given the relative recent establishment of the groupings and the transient nature of their respective memberships. They do, however, to varying degrees, address some of the informational, protection, and socio-emotional needs of their members.

Advantages of Enclaves

An enclave is a space that "offers a continuity of context" (Grinberg & Grinberg, 1982, p. 141), and the Africana networks in southern China and Shanghai can be considered enclaves in certain ways. It is a replication, to some degree, of important aspects of home within the host country. Its members provide empathy and understanding and therefore make the pain of loss and the anxieties of the new bearable. It ideally validates a sense of ongoing-being and continuity, even as the individual develops new coping strategies and modifies the sense of self with the goal of developing "an imaginative, creative attitude toward becoming assimilated into the new world around him" (Grinberg & Grinberg, p. 141). Important for members of these recent enclaves is the availability of real-time data on matters related to doing well in China and in managing risk. So, the enclave in southern China is a vital source of information on the protocols around trading successfully with the Chinese or negotiating interactions with Chinese administrators. While in Shanghai, where the network is an electronically mediated one, the focus is on sharing information on job opportunities, negotiating workplace challenges, and facilitating social life.

The enclave facilitates those seeking to assuage, to varying degrees, the sense of loss of the home. Such a space and function allow the foreigner to mourn, regroup, and take steps to adapt to the demands of the new culture (Grinberg & Grinberg, 1982). The enclave, however, is also the site of struggle between two longings: that for home and that for the host culture. Therefore, it ideally offers the possibility of a space within which one may not only mourn the loss of important aspects of home, but also renegotiate psychosocial space in the host country. The enclave assists individuals in managing the anxieties inherent in being away from home even as they revel in the sense of establishing an optimal distance from home (Akhtar, 1995).

"Failure to negotiate the distance between these self-representations results in two problematic outcomes of identity: ethnocentric withdrawal and counter phobic assimilation" (Akhtar, 1995, p. 1063). With ethnocentric withdrawal, there is a tight hold on the idealized image of home. There is always the risk of being too intimate with the maternal pull of the home culture as represented by the enclave and its social markers. As a defense against this, one could observe a speedy adoption of the host culture alongside the renunciation of the home culture. This is not a realistic option for the Africana person in China, given the obstacles to becoming assimilated.

The anxieties associated with distance, such as melancholy and the unavailability of home, differ by culture; in some cultures, migration—with its accompanying psychological cost—is normative, with support mechanisms in place that mute the pain of distance and loss that is experienced. In cultures where such support mechanisms are not operational, the immigrant has difficulty establishing the appropriate psychic distance and negotiating entry, however constrained, into the host culture.

Transitional Space

Ideally, the enclave should function as a transitional space: one that permits some continuity with home, facilitates substantive immersion in and identification with the new, and allows for the integration of both psychic investments within the immigrant. There should ideally be a working sense of "we-ness" and belonging to the new culture. The enclave as a transitional space is empathic, indulges nostalgia, and facilitates mourning, thereby making anxieties more manageable and supporting forays into the new society. It validates a sense of ongoing-being and continuity, even as one develops new coping strategies and modifies the sense of self with "an imaginative creative attitude toward being assimilated into the new world around him" (Grinberg & Grinberg, 1982, p. 141).

This way of thinking about an enclave as a transitional space providing optimal distance to negotiate mourning the loss of the original home, and embracing the new can be questioned in some cases. In the case of Africana persons in China, there is little likelihood of assimilating into Chinese society given the cultural wariness and administrative obstacles to doing so as manifested in the difficulty in attaining permanent residence status and the virtual impossibility of becoming a naturalized Chinese citizen. Given this lack of opportunity to assimilate and the reluctance to return home, Africana persons in China remain psychologically in an in-between space and must find adaptive ways of managing the self in that space. They must hold on to gratifying aspects of both their original home and also the gratifying aspects of being in China. At the same time, the Africana person must be cognizant of the limitations of both and accept the reality of never quite having a home that satisfies all needs for belonging and self-growth.

Space for Managing a Sense of In-Betweenness

This requires the individual working with others to create psychosocial spaces in China that assuage belonging needs. Such a space is neither transitional nor a launching pad to assimilation and the relinquishing of the original home. This space is a transition into managing the sense of in-between-ness and is achieved through the creation of local Africana networks, which are distinctly evident in southern China.

There is recognition of a tendency by many Chinese persons to define all Africana persons in a homogeneous manner. There is little substantive acknowledgement of cultural differences within the Africana ascription. This results in a de facto marginalization of within group differences. Many subjects noted that many Chinese people view all Africana persons as from Africa. Especially in southern China, where the Africana person is subject to high levels of surveillance, there was a need to develop a group response to such wholesale and often negative *othering* by state authorities. Facilitated by the Nigerians in Guangzhou, an umbrella organization was formed in 2007 that sought to first reflect the diversity of Nigerians in Guangzhou and the challenges they faced. Emma, who has been in China for over 20 years, founded the organization and continues to lead it:

> The Nigerians [in Guangzhou] had an election, and I became their leader. When people cry, I pay attention. We had no office, and I said we could not be an association without an office. So in 2007, using my own funds, I rented an office. I studied the conditions and problems facing the Nigerians in Guangzhou and worked hard to unite them. I formed an umbrella organization based on the states of Nigeria.

The organization carries out several functions, three of which will be discussed here. It does educational work with its members around how to manage the psychosocial demands of life in southern China. In this regard, the organization sponsors two sets of activities, one of which speaks to the challenges of parenting with a focus on responsible fathering and naming rights. Emma noted:

> I arranged a Nigerian–Chinese Family Forum in 2012 to discuss the issue of the deportation of Chinese men who had Chinese families. The family suffers. Over 100 "Nigerians own factories and are married to Chinese women and are doing well. Their children need a future. Nigerians stress family, it keeps you happy. Unhappiness will affect your business."

With regard to names, he also observed:

> There are cultural differences with the Chinese around family names. The children [of Nigerian–Chinese unions] are seen as foreigners. The children must have a Chinese name to have citizenship, but then they lose their Nigerian family name, and the Chinese family can claim the child any day. My son must have my name.

The group also engages in indigenous policing, which Emma explains as follows:

> We also try to stop Nigerians coming in to commit crimes. We created a team called Peace Keepers, as these people were making problems for everyone. Whatever apply to Nigerians apply to all Africans, as Chinese [in Guangzhou] think that all Africans are Nigerians as we are the largest group, so for any crime, they blame Nigerians. Our name is at stake.

The organization also advocates for the interests of Nigerians to the Chinese authorities. These tend to revolve around justice issues, such as fair treatment of its members who have become involved with law enforcement or immigration officials. There is also advocacy to business authorities to ease some of the onerous restrictions encountered by Africana businesspersons. Emma noted that these services are offered to all Africana persons regardless of national origin. Abdoul, a Guinean businessman and community leader, spoke to this inclusivity when he noted:

> It is better for us to organize under one umbrella organization: Association of African Communities in China. It is not formalized, but there are frequent contacts with each other. We try to coordinate on the decisions we present to the Chinese: An African is an African.

In addition to this pan-Africana grouping, there are more nation-based organizations, some quite large and others, small and informal. Abdoul is also the leader of the fairly large Guinean community and explained its origins and functions as follows:

> In 2004, the Guinean community started growing here, so I began to organize it by forming an organization: The Guinean Association in Guangzhou. Started with 1,500 [people], but are now around 500. Many are quasi-literate and operate on the edge of the law. [There are] low educational levels among the French-speaking Africans. [It is] much higher among the Nigerians and Ghanaians. [They

> are] mostly Muslims. [They] marry young and around a third bring their wives with them.

He goes on to note that:

> We needed to advocate and fight for the interests of our members, hence the organization. We provide mostly social services. Guineans are very attached to home, so they will not stay here unlike the Nigerians. We have naming services, we arrange for bodies to be returned home. The Chinese do not want foreigners to be buried here.

There are more intimate groupings such as that facilitated by Cibana, a banking consultant, originally from Burundi:

> The Association of Africans is an informal grouping of people who have been here for 10 years or more. We socialize together every 2–3 months. This allows our children to socialize. There are a lot of inter-cultural married couples. I also meet regularly with families from Burundi and Angola and with White families. I try to diversify my groups.

Cibana is especially sensitive to the socialization of Afro-Chinese children, given their experience of cultural in-between-ness. He notes that:

> I teach my children (who have a Chinese mother) about African culture, but I also teach them that Africa is the future, and so they must know the culture. A multicultural upbringing will give them more choices. They will not be prisoners of certain beliefs but will be multi-cultural global citizens. I will not choose their identity for them. I want them to belong to a big nation. They know their roots but Burundi is too small. They were born in China but are still called foreigner. As mixed children, they are neither Chinese nor African.

Within Africana Group Challenges

The risk of mono-ethnic groupings arises when they become the only location of substantive relationships. So, there is a risk of cultural isolation and narrowness of experience when the Africana person in China focuses only on investing in relationships within his own group.

Allaya, a 32-year-old trader from Mali, has an elementary school education and prefers to socialize only with his own people: “It is difficult. Business friends are ok; very difficult to have social friends. I don’t need it, I only need work friends. All of my (social) friends are from Mali.” One can observe a similar pattern among some Africana technocrats, who socialize only with persons from the West who speak English. Such relationships can have the unwitting effect of limiting the diversity of cultural exposure, leaving biases unchallenged, and the Africana person is at risk to think about the Chinese as a homogeneous grouping, often with negative ascriptions.

Within Africana community commonalities often mute but do not eliminate tensions between groups. Lama, a 29-year-old Guinean trader, was scathing in her contempt for the Nigerians, portraying them as exploitive in business relationships and disrespectful of women. Yet when a family member had serious problems with the police, she did not hesitate to call on Emma, the Nigerian community leader, and his organization to provide extensive assistance. Others, especially in the Shanghai cohort, have noted that as they become more familiar with Chinese culture, they draw less on Africana group resources.

Transience is a feature of all Africana networks in China, with attendant high turnover of members, given that many are on temporary assignments or engage in shuttle migration. Others who might consider settling permanently quickly come to the conclusion that such a wish is not feasible. Within their ranks are seasoned sojourners who have a history, often beginning in childhood of frequent transnational moves. Some had parents who were diplomats, or the family migrated from the original home country to a diaspora setting, as evidenced by Caribbean folks who grew up in the United Kingdom or the United States or Nigerians who also grew up in the United States. As adults they engage in a nomadic existence; as a consequence of this, home is wherever they are.

A sense of community is still important to these individuals, and they too have formed an umbrella organization, the Caribbean Association of China. Among its fluid membership are persons of Africana heritage in addition to Caucasians from the West and Chinese individuals with Western exposure. The organization serves as an information network and socializes its members into understanding and managing themselves in China. Within this group, there are rarely substantive visa renewal or criminal law enforcement issues. The group also provides cultural entertainment and familiarity in ways that are gratifying and not too demanding in terms of identity choices. They organize fund-raising galas around benign themes such as carnival and pirates, the proceeds of which go toward assisting disadvantaged Chinese children. The community in Shanghai faces a subtle but psychologically enervating risk in that given that many of its members work for international companies, their interactions are often mostly with Western-oriented Chinese persons. They reside in a cosmopolitan city and can therefore become fairly cocooned and indifferent to interacting with a diverse set of Chinese citizens. This cultural isolation is exacerbated by the fact that many do not speak Chinese, and therefore it heightens the sense of in-between-ness.

Community With the Chinese

A significant challenge for both the Shanghai and Guangzhou cohorts is managing their relationships with Chinese individuals across a range of areas. The issue of being Black in China will be discussed in the next chapter, but it is surprisingly not the predominant challenge that most Africana persons face in China. While not denying the reality of racism, many Africana persons stated that, at its worst, it seemed less ingrained compared to their experiences in the West. This they attributed to the fact that once you took the time to work on the relationship and the other person had good intentions, the issue of race receded. Lama's experience as trader was typical of many: "I have met more people so I have a better understanding of culture." This was unlike the West, where no matter how close the relationship, race was widely perceived to be always an issue.

For many Africana persons, there was a need to learn to tolerate widespread but un-hygienic Chinese habits such as indiscriminate spitting and coughing and the apparent widespread lack of the use of deodorant. Related to this was the pervasiveness of staring at persons of color, shoving, and sometimes occurrences of inappropriate touching, for instance a situation where a Chinese person would rub the skin of an Africana person to see if the Blackness would rub off. Many saw these behaviors as the cost of being in China, and they perceived that one had to adjust.

What was most striking for many was the capitalist nature of China. Kristina, a 46-year-old African American corporate trainer, observed:

> I am in a communist country, but it is the most capitalist place I have ever been. They perceive us [Americans] as having a social net. They feel they must work a lot to live well. They act as if they have never had anything; as if they are not used to anything.

Chips, a Nigerian American investor, noted with pleasure that, "There are always opportunities here. … It is the Wild West here, anything goes. … You can start any business anytime."

Cecilia, an investment advisor, notes that: "I think [money] is what drives this country. The government holds shares in everything. People are into money so will sell fake anything. I have never seen people who like money more than the Chinese." She goes on to note, "It is a good place to be. It is right. You are welcomed. You are not drained out simply because you are Black. You feel equal to anyone else."

Thomas, a 39-year-old entrepreneur of French and Malian heritage, spoke to the personal agency that this capitalist culture afforded the foreigner:

> There is equal opportunity here. No matter if you are Black, Brown, Indian, or Jew, as long as you work, in Shanghai they like you. Equal

> opportunity is Shanghai. If Blacks went to a club, then the Chinese followed. Blacks could make or break the club.

Needless to say, there were also less complimentary observations about Chinese culture, one of which—challenges around being innovative—has provided a market niche for the Africana technocrats working and living in China. Bill, the informal teacher of English, summarized this as follows, "They think, but they don't dream." He went on to note that, "They don't think outside the box; they are locked in the box. They are grounded on earth locked in day-to-day living. No time to think."

Wei Wei, the real estate executive, attributes such caution to a fear of losing face:

> If it is not written on paper they are not going to do it. Do not ask them to go off script. Do not ask them to think. They will try to be flexible if it does not make them lose face. My ballet teacher will faithfully and quickly pick up a technique. They will not express themselves. They tend to devalue their own work by saying things like, "I am not good at it."

William, a 35-year-old shoe designer who is originally from the Bahamas and who was recruited in the United States to work in China, commented on this issue of initiative:

> Their model is to copy not to create so I knew I could make money here. They were surprised that I could create a design for a shoe rather than just copy. So China was where I could make the final money.

He noted that he was committed to facilitating innovative thinking on the part of his Chinese workers and would encourage his assistant to express her opinions and to share her ideas. He was however taken aback when she informed him that her task was not to think but to carry out his ideas. Some argued that this reluctance spoke to a fear that taking chances could be risky for their well-being and that many Chinese people, while quite creative, thought it best to keep a low profile; they did not want attention.

Nevertheless, beneath this apparent caution was a hunger for knowledge on the part of many Chinese persons; many Africana persons felt that this hunger added a false quality to their relationship with some Chinese people. There was a perception that once they knew you were knowledgeable, they would cultivate a relationship, glean as much knowledge as possible, and then lose interest in you. Jay, the Congolese banker with many years of interacting with the Chinese, gave a quite nuanced view of this challenge: "He will be your friend if he can get what he wants from you. Once he gets that it stops. You will have few friends based on just liking you. This is also true of their own Chinese-Chinese relationships." Jay, who is fluent in Chinese and has lived there for decades, has also developed gratifying and sustained relationships with Chinese citizens. Being fluent in Chinese and cultivating social, non-business relationships over time appears to be the common thread among Africana persons engaged in enduring and gratifying relationships with Chinese persons. They are the ones who have close Chinese friends, have visited their homes, and have been adopted by their families. By way of contrast, those who do not speak Chinese and engage in only business relationships tend to have the more jaundiced view. This is especially evident with Africana people in the cutthroat, low-trust trading culture of Guangzhou.

Ethics

A consistent theme for many of the subjects was the challenge around ethical relating with many business Chinese persons. Individuals in China finds themselves increasingly in a sociopolitical space that grants a bounded autonomy seemingly less tied to moral strictures (Kleinman et al., 2011). Such an individual is encouraged to be productive, an important benefit of which is the reaping of cognitive and material rewards in a marketplace that can be quite amoral. As a consequence, much energy must be devoted to negotiating and being vigilant around ethical issues. Harry, an entrepreneur, spoke to the importance of ethical discipline:

> This is the new El Dorado. You can be wronged very easily here because it is new. But even if you have solid foundations you must assess yourself because you can get caught up in the doing, lose your values, misunderstand the limits. You must be careful who you do things with and how you do things.

The Africana person is ideally able to observe commonalities and differences across categories: The insight that such observation yields in turn facilitates a more discerning and ethically responsible approach to ongoing self-work and to relating. This speaks to vigilance and ongoing discourse with regard to when to be flexible and when to stand firm in relation to self in the world. A good-enough understanding of the basis of subjective yearnings and imperatives in relation to an ethical stance is helpful here.

There is a sense among some that the pursuit of wealth by the Chinese drives much of the unethical behavior observed. Elaine's observation was fairly typical: "Money is their God. Their moral compass is out of sync. There is a lot of corruption and there does not appear to be much concern if someone is hurt." One therefore hears of numerous incidents of being swindled, with Jocelyn's trading encounter being fairly typical:

> I have a lot of disappointment in my (Chinese) business partners. I helped them and trusted them, and they robbed me. I know more about friendship now. Myself and another guy from Togo worked with a Chinese man in Guangzhou. We generated a lot of money, but he did not pay me, so I left after 9 months. He was not happy as the customers trusted me. Many of the customers came with me when I left.

There was a sense that especially between private individuals, contracts would not necessarily be honored and quality was an ongoing challenge.

Many argued that this state of affairs existed in part due to the weak system of fair accountability, within which there was bias against the foreigner, the rules were opaque and fluid, and communication was difficult. Lama, whose family member was arrested, complained that, "They arrest you but find nothing but they still keep you. You have no rights, you cannot talk. If they accuse you, you cannot defend yourself."

Given such scenarios, one is tempted to think that China has no contemporary moral history given the prohibition on publically discussing prominent ethical struggles such as the Cultural Revolution, the student appeals in Tiananmen Square and the attendant pain. These events were costly on the individual and group level and continue to exert influence on the culture, but they are not part of the permissible public debate as to how China builds a productive and just society in a neoliberal and globalized world (Kleinman et al., 2011). One cost to the individual is an awareness of the history of struggle that must be borne silently, even as the elites make seemingly ethical appeals to inform individual behavior. In the interest of a shallow harmony, the pain and associated political difficulties of past struggles for an ethical society can neither be named nor discussed (Kleinman et al., 2011).

The ethical landscape is not without its attractive features. Both the Chinese and the Africana communities share a human capability to relate and come from respective histories of an ethics grounded in strong affective ties despite ideological and administrative challenges. These challenges give rise to ambivalence that if handled adaptively strengthens the groups and their members.

Emma, the Nigerian community leader, interacts a lot with the Chinese authorities and noted the following: "If you respect them and their system it shows you respect yourself and that gives them face and they will try to assist you and that gives you face." Given the weak formal structures of ethical accountability, personal relationships are an important means by which to ensure one is treated fairly. This means doing the work of learning the language and investing in relationships. Harry spoke to this work:

> You have to gain the trust of the Chinese, but most foreigners stick to their own and don't make an attempt to learn Chinese culture. The Chinese know this and so keep their distance. I am not like that; feel like I was Chinese in my previous life.

Others reported having enduring relationships with not only a Chinese individual but also with their families.

Ethical projects are sustained by the individual being embedded in relationships that temper personal imperatives by calling upon those in the relationship to be sensitive to each other's needs. This is challenging given that for many Africana persons in China, there is not always a commitment to understanding the ethical landscape in which they are embedded. To adapt in an ethically informed way, they must be sensitive to seeming differences that when examined require toleration or mask substantive commonalities.

Some differences can be embraced, and others must be rejected in the context of being sensitive to implicit biases. Such work requires Africana people in China to avoid a shallow toleration anchored to condescension or limited to intellectualization, bereft of any affective connection (Bauman, 1991). They must, at times, be able to tolerate an irreducible otherness of the *other* that cannot be understood and ought not to be demonized or denigrated in a narcissistic pursuit of transparency or in the grip of a sense of moral superiority. This is a daunting ethical agenda given that the average Africana person in China often lacks a command of the Chinese language, which in turn makes it difficult to develop and sustain interdependent relationships that are not market mediated.

Adaptive Ambivalence

As noted in previous sections, the Africana individual must find healthy ways of managing ambivalence. Following are some illustrations of approaches to doing so, some of which are gratifying and others of which speak to some eating of bitterness.

Pleasure in Achievement

The insightful Africana person in China becomes increasingly aware of the need to celebrate the pleasures of being in China derived from an embrace of the opportunities it offers for self-development and resource acquisition. Fueling the move to China is a curiosity that is often evident in those who voluntarily leave their homelands and might also speak to dissatisfaction with the stasis and immobility of home. There is an orientation toward difference manifested as an interest in fresh perspectives that is challenging to the standard ways of viewing the world (Grinberg & Grinberg, 1982). Such a stance not only disrupts the normative and its constraining ethos, but also orients the individual away from nostalgia and toward fashioning a new self-agenda (Headley, 2011).

Alongside curiosity is a capacity to tolerate difference and, as mentioned above, to be open to experiences that are disruptive to established ways of thinking. Thus Elaine spoke of her initial surprise at drinking hot water as opposed to cold water but quickly adjusted to the practice and later embraced the practice when she read about its purported medicinal benefits. Such toleration is also facilitated by living in Chinese communities, as Elaine does, where difference is the norm and her own cultural practices are considered alien. Again, the challenge is to know when to adapt, when to reject, and when to hold both in tension. So, Wei Wei quickly learned Chinese and developed a substantial and sustained relationship with a Chinese woman. At the same time, she rejected her advice that she needed to cloister herself at home for weeks following the birth of her child.

So, with many Africana persons, there was a sense of pleasure at discovering heretofore unrecognized talents and various new ways of asserting the self. Such derived pleasures were often understood within the context of the lack of resources or undue restrictions in the home country. The thrust toward self-improvement speaks to the practice of *suzhi*, but with a greater focus on self as against self-improvement in the service of the nation.

Emeline is a 27-year-old French woman of Guadeloupian heritage who grew up in both Guadeloupe and France. She has a postgraduate degree and has been living in China for the past 3 years working as a business executive. Before coming to China she lived in Brazil. She described her development in China as follows:

> My mind is more open, I see less boundaries. In China, everything is possible. In China, if you want to do something you just do it. In 3 years, I became sales manager with a team of 10 foreigners. My friends at home would not have done this so fast. I have matured much faster. Thinking about doing investments in France would be more constrained. I have moved much faster here. I would have been constrained in France. In France, I would not have thought about investing, and the knowledge would have been harder to get.

For some, the emphasis was on intellectual achievements; Jay noted that he had attained two academic degrees in China, while others like Yoda and Wei Wei took pride in their mastery of Chinese. Then there was the sense of having achieved a desired level of economic achievement, with

Lama, a trader, noting, "I am a better businessperson. Buy one item here in China and sell it for the price of two in Africa." Others spoke to remittances to home to support family and to invest in property.

Pleasurable Otherness

An often-overlooked aspect of otherness that was noted by many Africana persons in China was the admiration of the skill sets they brought to or developed in China. Not only was there the pleasure derived from being paid well, but there was also the interest in them demonstrated by the Chinese.

Ann is a 29-year-old Jamaican woman with a master's degree in politics from a Chinese university and now teaches English to adults and children. She has been in China for the past 3 years and prior to coming to China worked at various administrative jobs in Jamaica.

> I found them warm and loving. I was invited to the home of a family and they treated me nicely; felt genuine. I teach their kids so not always sure (about how genuine they are), but they are always willing to help even strangers.

Cecilia and others spoke about the necessity of working hard to develop relationships:

> Because of their culture, they do not talk to anyone before they know you. Neighbors take a long time to talk to you. They need to know, "Who are you? Why are you here?" This is also the same in their Chinese relationships. They do not answer questions directly.

As noted earlier in this chapter, many interviewees shared with me that this pleasure in having one's skills validated comes at a cost. Many observed that one must simply adapt to the casual racism such as the preference for White foreigners, the increased cost for services, and the difficulty in engaging Chinese peers to socialize outside of work. This speaks to the constant reminders that the individual is a foreigner and must be kept at a distance.

Irreducible Identifications

In the traditional psychological model of migration, there was little possibility of return, so acceptance of loss through mourning would eventually reduce the need to engage in splitting over time (Grinberg & Grinberg, 1982). Psychological investments in home would be withdrawn and invested in the new adopted home country. For the Africana person, there is ambivalence, as it would be risky to emotionally invest in the idea of China as a permanent home given its antipathy toward the foreigner and unwelcoming immigration regime. The original home therefore remains a site of ambivalence, with its pleasures and frustrations in tension with each other but still an important internalized site for a sense of validated belonging. Staying in touch through electronic media and visiting home, which is facilitated by relatively inexpensive transportation, results in the Africana person often holding home in an in-between place of desire, gratification, and disappointment. The ambivalence ensures that while there is painful awareness of home's shortcomings, there can be no wholesale condemnation of home given its historical self-forming gratifications. The sense of belonging that would provide such gratifications in China cannot be substantially developed in the absence of Chinese language fluency, and the restrictions on the possibility of permanent residence. One hears frequent lamentations from Africana persons about the sense of always being an outsider no matter how long they have lived in China.

The ambivalence is also sustained by identification with home that might be based on psychological constructions of home and of China that are at a remove from the social realities of those sites. So, while for many the home in the head is fueled by both memories and contact with the realities of home, for others, there may be less contact and more using of the memories as a base for the construction of a fantastical but gratifying sense of home. Such a strategy acts as a basis for a reassuring sense of belonging and as a buffer against the narcissistic injuries incurred by the rejection of overtures to make China home. Grinberg and Grinberg (1982) capture the foreigner's task as follows:

> At the same time that I confronted the problem of maintaining my identity I struggled to change it, because when I de-idealized my task, I could accept the "bad" aspects of my old culture and incorporate the "good" aspects of the new without completely renouncing my previous identifications.
>
> (p. 164)

In summary, for Africana persons to be successful in China, there can be no complete relinquishing of home; neither can there be a substantive embracing of China as the new home.

Reflective Style

The individual who leaves the home country is, to some degree, skeptical of the norm, curious about difference, and perhaps comfortable with a reflective process. The identifications of individuals like this, while influenced by ethnicity, race, and other primordial markers, are more closely wedded to self-competencies such as technical skills and critical reasoning abilities (Strenger, 2013). They tend to privilege cognitively oriented performance outcomes as the metric of success. Many Africana persons, as noted earlier, were justly proud of their intellectual achievements and material acquisitions. This approach confronts the Africana person with two significant dilemmas. The first of these is the psychological effort necessary to maintain high levels of productivity. This is especially demanding in a market culture that requires frequent, in-depth thought about how and when one challenges deep-seated traditional practices that seek to limit one's innovative approach. So, the attractiveness of China, in its seeming desire for innovative foreigners, is stymied by traditional ways of doing business that created the need for this type of creative worker in the first place. Africana people must be reflective as to how they can be innovative in a culture that is ambivalent about innovation. So, while there is success in doing their jobs, they must reflect on how to manage the frustrations of being stymied and how to be innovative in culturally tolerated ways.

The second dilemma is the realization that Africana workers' need for a sense of themselves as successful that is initially linked to the market, and to measurable success, is soon assuaged. This gives rise to other needs that are not as easily satisfied, and issues of community, spirituality, sexuality, and intimacy can be an ongoing challenge for them.

Such thoughtfulness requires a reflective style that is sensitive to the need to devote resources to exploring and enjoying other aspects of life. In that regard, there are aspects of Chinese culture that have proven helpful for Africana persons interested in exploring ways of being and aesthetic appreciations that are not market driven. One person reported immersing herself more in Buddhist practices, to enable her to developer a holistic understanding of herself, given her current overly materialistic lifestyle. Another Africana person has embarked on a systemic exploration of Eastern Asia given low transportation costs and ease of travel.

One ironic outcome of these initiatives is a subtle change in reflective style that blurs the tendency of some Africana persons to dichotomize East and West and allows them in turn to be able to tolerate multiple perspectives on a given situation. Raoul from Guadeloupe made the following observation:

> [I am] more open minded. I have a wider perspective and I am more tolerant. I have grown intellectually and as a musician. I work harder at trying to understand; to be less aggressive. I must feel good about China, must relate. I have fewer stereotypes about the Chinese.

This capacity to observe and selectively embrace the local as part of their reflective approach is psychologically gratifying, but also costly for Africana people. They must hold the differences that are truly different in productive tension with deep commonalities across the culture divide. One Africana woman from the Caribbean related to me, in a rather bemused manner, a conversation with a Chinese friend on this issue. She had trotted out her distaste for the idea of eating dog meat. Her Chinese friend had laughed and pointed out to her that most Chinese do not eat dog meat and that many Caribbean people eat goat, frog, crocodile, and the face of the cow, culinary preferences that she would never entertain. They both laughed. This quality of reflection is often necessary given that the Africana person is constantly working the commonality/difference boundary.

The Africana individual is constantly thinking about when to tolerate, when to embrace, and when to resist. This is challenging because, given that there is a social component to being reflective, thought must be given as who one choses to do such work with. For Africana persons who are fluent in Chinese, there is access to a larger pool of persons willing to engage in such work.

Relationships between members of the Africana community in China also highlight commonalities and differences to be celebrated in some cases and tolerated in others. For many Africana persons from the West, this was their first sustained exposure to Africans from the continent. Facilitated in part by the Chinese tendency to perceive them as a homogeneous grouping, many reveled in the commonality of experiences alongside an appreciation of the diverse ways in which one could be an Africana person. Beyond pride in Blackness, which is explored in the next chapter, was a realization of the self as able to grow and at the same time have some aspects be validated as positive. Some Africana women from the West, while finding some aspects of the relationship gratifying, were often quite disapproving of what they saw as archaic masculine positions on gender relations by Africana men across the geographical spectrum.

Resilience

For the Africana person, there is a need to be resilient in the face of the need to eat bitterness, to accept that some self-goals will never come to fruition in China. So, individuals must be pragmatic in the face of both petty and substantive institutionalized antipathy toward the foreigner. Such accommodation is emotionally costly but in the short-to-medium term is a part of the cost of being a foreigner and being Black in China. Garba, from Mali, spoke to his coping strategy:

> There are a lot of negative stereotypes regarding Africa in China; less educated, going against the social norms. You must have a high standard of social conduct; be the best you can be; be dignified as the Chinese value this. Do not live the negative stereotype.

Oftentimes, the pursuit of a goal central to the Africana's person's well-being, such as spirituality, can be quite daunting and requires resilience in the face of the need to eat bitterness. As a consequence, many persons report that they found the officially sanctioned churches theologically bland and spiritually unsatisfying, given the state requirement that homilies be free of social commentary. This lack has given rise to underground churches that offer more inspiring sermons but are always at risk of being shut down (Haugen, 2012). One Africana person who asked not to be identified described the process as follows:

> We often rented space in a night club on a Sunday morning and would have our services. After a while, the public security people would text us to desist, and then we would move to another site and the whole process would start again.

She reported that while this process was not only irritating and risky, it strengthened her religious beliefs and that the harassment was part of the cost of spiritual uplift. Others spoke of being more tolerant and learning to accept some differences as being unassailable and therefore something one had to accommodate to. John, from Uganda, noted:

> I have gotten very better at controlling my temper; I use to be impatient, anxious. I thought things could be just the way I wanted it. I learned that if I was patient and focused I would get what I wanted. I also learned to be more self-reliant.

Such insight speaks to the deployment of an adaptive stance that while generating some ambivalence is a necessary compromise.

Limits on Splitting

The Africana person must manage judiciously the emotional response toward home that animates activity in China, given that it is a source of both pleasure and longing alongside disappointment and flight. In the traditional psychoanalytic model of migration, splitting was an understandable way of managing the loss of home (Akhtar, 1995). Splitting refers to the difficulty in holding simultaneously in consciousness both positive and negative emotional feelings toward an issue or person. To resolve the conflict, the individual must perceive the person or issue as either good or bad, but not both. That which is bad, in this case home, is distanced from, and over time there is less emotional investment in it. In addition, its shortcomings are emphasized with a concomitant privileging of the gratifications derived in the host country that would eventually become the new home.

While there is some splitting among some Africana persons in China, it is more muted given that many harbor strong positive feelings of home and entertain possibilities of eventually returning there—possibilities that are realistic for some. For others, there might be no ultimate desire to return, but there is considerable investment in home from the perspective of a valued internalized identity base, and therefore, aspects of home are treasured. This is crucial for many a modern foreigner residing temporarily in a host country that refuses to allow it to be used as a site of a new identity and home.

Managing Aloneness

This sense of in-between-ness, where identity and not-quite-belonging coexist, is emotionally costly, requiring a robust capacity to manage the attendant, and, at times, painful emotional states (Grinberg & Grinberg, 1982), that arise from being in a cultural space that is limited in its willingness to make the Africana person fully a part of the host community. This will resonate with a related aloneness in the home country given its inability to accommodate to some of the individual's self-strivings. For the successful Africana person, the crucial legacy of home is a good-enough emotional sense of self as loved and as belonging despite dissatisfactions with the group, where those dissatisfactions do not involve a sense of being violated or fundamentally rejected.

It is that irreducible sense of belonging that allows the Africana person to be in a place like China that withholds that possibility of substantive inclusion and validation of the Africana person's need to belong. Put another way, the Africana person who enters China with an established and positive sense of belonging is able to tolerate the sense of otherness experienced at home and in China. The paradox here is that the sense of aloneness is better managed and allows for adaptive ambivalence, providing that the core experience of home was a benign and loving one, despite its inevitable shortcomings. It allows the individual to maintain a psychological stance of accepting the pain of not-quite-belonging, while at the same time embracing opportunities for growth.

Grinberg and Grinberg (1982) argue that there is a defensive aspect to this position, as the individual must accept that she or he is not an immigrant, that there will never be full acceptance into the host community, and that resources must be devoted to managing this painful aspect of being, to some degree, eternally other. A methodological observation is pertinent here. I obviously interviewed subjects who have stayed in China and for the most part perceive themselves as having done well there. I did not interview persons who left China, some of whom might well have found the aloneness and the sense of exclusion emotionally too costly a price to pay.

The Africana person in China has experiences that are quite varied; these experiences are mediated, in part, by the intellectual and emotional resources that individuals had developed prior to coming to China. In addition, the quality of the support groups—at home, in the diaspora, and in China—from the perspectives of knowledge and contacts also influence the ability of Africana foreign workers to achieve their desired outcomes. Central to being successful is the capacity of the individual to effectively manage the ambivalence experienced about the home country and being in China. They must come to terms with experiencing good-enough well-being, while existing in an in-between psychological space, accepting the reality of not being fully at home, whether in their original home country or in China.

References

Adams, C. J. (2015). Structure and agency: Africana immigrants in China. *Journal of Pan African Studies*, *7*(10), 85–108.

Akhtar, S. (1995). A third individuation: Immigration, identity and the psychoanalytic process. *Journal of the American Psychoanalytic Association*, *43*(4), 1051–1084.

Akyeapong, E. (2000). Africans in the diaspora: The diaspora of Africa. *African Affairs*, *99*, 193–215.

Bauman, Z. (1991). *Modernity and ambivalence*. London, UK: Polity Press.

Beltsiou, J. (2016). Seeking home in the foreign: Otherness and immigration. In J. Beltsiou (Ed.), *Immigration in psychoanalysis* (pp. 89–108). New York, NY: Routledge.

Bodomo, A. (2010). The African trading community in Guangzhou: An emerging bridge for Africa-China relations. *The China Quarterly*, *203*, 693–707.

Bodomo, A. (2012). *Africans in China*. Amherst, NY: Cambria Press.

Castillo, R. (2015). Homing' Guangzhou: Emplacement, belonging and precarity among Africans in China. *International Journal of Cultural Studies*, *18*(2), 1–20.

Castillo, R. (2016). How many Africans are in Guangzhou? Retrieved from https://africansinchina.net/how-many-africans-are-there-in-guangzhou/

Castles, S. (2010). Understanding global migration: A social transformative perspective. *Journal of Ethnic and Migration Studies*, *36*(10), 1565–1586.

de Haas, H. (2014). Migration theory: Quo Vadis? (DEMIG project paper 24, University of Oxford: International Migration Institute).

Dikotter, F. (1992). *The discourse of race in modern China*. London, UK: Hurst & Company.

Echeruo, M. (1999). An African diaspora: The ontological project. In I. Okpewho, C. Davies, & A. Mazrui (Eds.), *The African diaspora* (pp. 3–18). Bloomington, IN: Indiana University Press.

Edwards, N. (2005). Diaspora, difference and Black internationalisms. *Small Axe*, *9*(1), 120–128.

Fennell, V. (2013). Race: China's question and problem. *Review of Black Political Economy*, *40*, 245–275.

Gallicchio, M. (2000). *The African American encounter with Japan and China: Black internationalism in Asia, 1895–1945*. Chapel Hill, NC: University of North Carolina Press.

Grinberg, L., & Grinberg, R. (1982). *Psychoanalytic perspectives on migration and exile*. New Haven, CT: Yale University Press.

Hall, S. (1990). Cultural identity and diaspora. In J. Rutherford (Ed.), *Identity, community, culture and difference* (p. 234). London, UK: Lawrence & Wishart. Retrieved from www.rlwclarke.net/Theory/SourcesPrimary/HallCulturalIdentityandDiaspora.pdf

Haugen, H. (2012). Nigerians in China: A second state of immobility. *International Migration*, *50*(2), 65–80.

Haugen, H. (2015). Destination China: The country adjusts to its new migration reality. Retrieved from http://migrationpolicy.org/article/destination-china-country-adjusts-its-new-migration-reality

Headley, C. (2011). George Lamming and the epistemology of exile: Ways of seeing, singularity and colonialism. In A. Bogues (Ed.), *The George Lamming reader: The aesthetics of decolonialisation* (pp. 287–310). Kingston, Jamaica: Ian Randle Publishers.

Kleinman, A., Yan, Y., Jun, J., Lee, S., Zhang, E., Tianshu, P., … Jinhau, G. (Eds.). (2011). *Deep China: The moral life of the person: What anthropology and psychiatry tell us about China today*. Berkeley, CA: University of California Press.

Morais, I. (2009). Chinese "Wahala": The tribulations of Nigerian "Bushfallers" in a Chinese territory. *Journal of Global Cultural Studies*, *5*, 2–22.

Pinheiro, F., & Chaplin, I. (2015). Africans in Macau. Retrieved from http://documents.mx/documents/africans-in-macao.html

Raijman, R. (2012). Foreigners and outsiders: Exclusionist attitudes toward labor migrants in Israel. *International Migration*, *51*(2), 136–151.

Sen, A. (1989). Development as capability expansion. *Journal of Development Planning*, *19*, 41–58.

Skeldon, R. (2012). China: An emerging destination for economic migration. Retrieved from www.migrationinformation.org/Profiles/display.cfm?ID=838

Strenger, C. (2013). The new cosmopolitans: Challenges and discontents. *Psychoanalytic Psychology*, *30*(2), 264–280.

Torres-Saillant, S. (2009). One and divisible: Mediations on global Blackness. *Small Axe*, *29*(13), 4–25.

Wang, F. (2010). China's population destiny: The looming crisis. *Current history*. Retrieved from http://search.proquest.com/docview/749603801?pq-origsite=gscholar

7 Africana Persons and Self-Making in China

It is in China many African persons are confronted with the fact that they are perceived as Black and not necessarily in a positive light. This requires an investment in doing identity work, teasing out the many ways to be Black and when to deploy a particular variant. This also requires rethinking and often re-signifying the negatively tinged models of Blackness that were a function of being socialized in the home country with colonial legacies.

Vignette: About Dean

Dean, a 27-year-old gay Bahamian man with an undergraduate degree from a Chinese university, has lived in Shanghai for the past 5 years. He is a partner in a company that exports industrial goods to the Caribbean, and prior to that, he taught English language skills to Chinese students. Dean has a good working knowledge of the Chinese language and can read and speak with a good degree of fluency—such competency being a prerequisite for foreigners to study in a Chinese university—and this accomplishment has, importantly, allowed him to form more substantive relationships with people from China.

Dean's parents both died when he was quite young, but he remembers his grandparents as a source of strength and guidance: "I remember as a child feeling lonely. … [I] would be sad. My grandmother never made you feel you were any less a person than the other kids. So despite the loss I felt, I was a person of worth." When he was a young adult, a teacher in the Bahamas implored Dean to leave:

> I had a Jamaican teacher and she threatened me: "Get out, go abroad and get a university education." She saw my strengths. I could write. She pushed me and stayed on me. She would not accept mediocrity. She said that I had the mentality of an old person, that I was wise beyond my years.

While the external motivation for leaving came directly from Dean's teacher, internally Dean struggled with his sexual identity—specifically, the difficult and fraught experience of living as a self-identified gay man in the Caribbean, where there is often much homophobia. "I always knew I did not fit in at home. I am a gay man and that comes with a lot of discrimination along with verbal and physical abuse," he said.

Language, Identity, Racism, and Construction of Blackness in China

Dean initially had no specific interest in going to China, but he was inclined to seek a foreign locale where he could safely and productively work on further understanding and developing himself. His interest in and subsequent move to China was facilitated by a friend who had recently returned to China after a vacation at home: "He convinced me to come and try it out. I had a plan and China was not in it but I took a risk."

Dean initially found China both exhilarating and daunting:

> I came to China without expectations, and it was an eye-opener; the pointing, the staring, whispering in my face. I had to rethink for the first time in my adult life: Who are you? Are you comfortable with who you are? I had to learn to be myself but also to be respectful with [others]; not get pissed off or disgruntled because they did not understand who they were looking at. I think they perceived me the way I would have if I were in their shoes.

Dean's mandatory 10-month intensive Chinese language program helped with working on these thoughts and feelings. As a consequence of his competency in speaking Chinese, Dean was able to form substantive relationships with persons from China, remarking that "I felt comfortable when I started to learn the language, and I was able to have really good relationships with Chinese friends."

But Dean still had to navigate his sense and experience of Blackness in China. According to Dean, the meaning and value he attached to race was quite complex and evolved over time. Initially, he felt unprepared to deal with racism, sharing these remarks:

> I did not quite fit in when I went to China as I had poor self-esteem; it was very bad. I was not sure of myself. There was this battle to figure out who I am; what I should be doing. Being in China meant two battles, one of which was a lifelong battle. Going to China was not just another part of that battle but the biggest as I also had to deal with racism and that does not exactly help your self-esteem. Living in China helped me to win that battle. China built my self-confidence. I am more in tune with my Blackness; not having to doubt my Blackness.

The challenge for Dean was to rethinking his cultural identity partly within the context of confronting racism.

Social Interaction

Crucial for Dean's psychosocial evolution was his ability to find diverse social spaces to tease out the nuances of Blackness and to observe commonalities within difference. In his interactions with Chinese friends, for example, he observed:

> I had a lot of Chinese friends who would tell me that I am brown; not really Black compared to the dark-skinned Africans. Given my relationships with my African friends I told my Chinese friends that while the Africans look different than me we are not really different; we are really the same.

Among Dean's African friends, issues of his Blackness were also contested in a way that was interpreted as good-natured:

> I had friends from Kenya and Libya, and they would tease me and laugh at me, saying that I was not really Black because I had White blood that made me brown. I was always curious about Africans, and being in China was my first opportunity to really get to know them and have them as friends. China was my first time to eat, party, and think with them; to really get to know them.

Dean was also able to become quite comfortable with his Blackness in the context of feeling confident, competent, and able to represent and educate others, specifically Chinese persons:

> I was looking for a job, and in China, it is common practice to send in your photo with your application; that way they can see your race. If you are Black you almost never get a call to come in. For some reason, this company did not ask for a photo but simply scheduled me for an interview. When I walked in, they simply stared, and it was clear to me that I was not what they expected. Shock. Amazement. What's this guy here for? From that moment, I knew I was going to have to blow these folks away. I was already fluent in Mandarin, so I answered all the questions in Mandarin. Before I left, they offered me the position. I had to break down the barriers of their perceptions of Blackness; violent, poor, and illiterate. Even when I was on campus, they looked at us differently to how they looked at Whites. The Whites were the ideal employees; they were viewed as professionals. I had to do my best to show them that people of color could be the same.

Discussion

In this vignette, some core themes emerge around the experience of being Black in China. One can observe sensitivity to issues of belonging alongside a sense of being other at home. Dean grew up in a primarily Afro-Caribbean culture and was exposed to diverse models of striving, some of whom were of successful persons who were proud of their Africana heritage. At the same time, his home country felt economically limiting in the opportunities, it could provide in facilitating personal development and was sexually oppressive.

This mix of ethnic and cultural pride and economic limitation created for Dean an internalized sense of ambivalence: his home was suffused in love and provided positive recognition and belonging, he also felt strongly the effects of several structural constraints that placed real and significant limits on the possibilities for self-development. These structural shortcomings have led to the development and use of migration networks that facilitate entry into Canada the United States and parts of Europe; there is now a recently developing one in China.

Dean's experiences in China as an Africana resident have resulted in many new ways of thinking about Blackness and identity—some positive and some negative, some conscious and many unconscious as relates to race and geography. Such reflective work is further bolstered by him being embedded in groups of peers who represent diverse and positive ways of being Black. Dean's willingness to do such work helps him to clarify and appreciate the privileges and costs of being Black in China.

Achieving a Black identity that one can comfortably inhabit involves much self-work. Such achievement reflects a capacity to manage the tension between positive Black subjectivities that, as internalized representations, can sometimes involve unexamined notions of being Black. This alongside the complexities and challenges of the real-world experiences of often negative ascriptions about Blackness that can limit one's aspirations and sense of agency.

Some persons of Africana heritage report being socialized in Africana cultures where positive Blackness is taken as a given (Asante, 1993) or where, at best, Blackness is a category that serves as a lightly interrogated but positive component of self and identity. It is through the encounter with the other, in crossing the boundaries between Africana heritage and other cultures and spaces, that a reexamination of what it means to be Black in a non-Black space is often precipitated. The resulting reflective work can lead to different individual construction of Blackness.

The Africana person in China, by virtue of his noticeable physical differences, and in the context of the ambivalence directed at him by others, must constantly clarify, ideally through dialogue with others, what it means to be Black. Finally, such a resilient and well-grounded sense of

Blackness, along with the built-in flexibility necessary for cross-cultural migration, supports the work of self-development that first motivated the Africana person to live in China. It speaks to adaptively managing the ambivalence that results from experiencing both the attraction and aversion that come with being Black in China. As Dean's story demonstrates, adaptively managing these conflictual aspects of the self is one crucial practice that, for the Africana person, correlates with success in China.

Adaptive Ambivalence and Its Management

The perception of the Africana person in China offered by others is both varied and multiply determined. As a function of Blackness one may be admired, viewed warily, and also denigrated. An individual must hold these intense and oftentimes conflicting views together in tension and find an adaptive way to manage the ambivalence they give rise to. This is part of the work of self-development.

Yoda, a 32-year-old Africana school counselor, has resided in China for 6 years. He has lived in numerous countries as both a child and adult and is married with two children. Yoda has a benign view of the Chinese. He thinks that through the media they are exposed to both positive and negative images of Blackness and that this, combined with direct contact with African people, will result in them having a more positive and nuanced view.

> (Racism is) Not as strong here. The racism brings you together in the United States and Europe. Here you are a foreigner and a Black. There is no differentiation if you are a foreigner. The foreigner classification is strong. There is no felt racism here, more about ignorance.

Here, doing adaptive work requires understanding the impact of cultural forces on the self, while at the same time having some appreciation of one's identity and style of responding. Assisting in this work is being embedded in diverse cultural relationships that is supportive of the Africana person's identity work.

Multiplicity of Blackness

Relationship to Africa

There are myriad ways of defining Blackness, and at best, these ideas share two weak but enduring commonalities. The first of these is a perceived relationship to Africa—in our present story, this would imply that the Africana persons residing in China must come directly from various

African countries. In reality, the commonality can be quite weak: Group members directly from Africa do not define themselves as Africans or Black, preferring instead to anchor their identity claims in a nation (Mali), or an ethnic group (Yoruba). When asked, people have diverse ways to describe their racial and ethnic identities, and the following are but three of the examples that I heard that can offer a glimpse of the amazing diversity in understanding the term *Blackness* among Africana persons born on the continent of Africa living in China.

Abdoul is a 61-year-old Guinean with a postgraduate degree in economics, who has lived in varied locales in Africa and has had substantive commercial links with China for nearly 30 years. He has resided in Guangzhou with his Guinean wife since 2003, and they have three children. Abdoul owns and manages a trading company that exports goods to various African countries. Prior to moving to Guangzhou, he worked for many years as a government procurement officer and then as the head of his own company importing industrial equipment. He became interested in China when his customers complained about the cost of European equipment relative to Chinese-manufactured equivalents.

Abdoul is unequivocal in his affirmation of his Blackness:

> I have always been proud of my Blackness. I refused to take the French nationality. I was entitled to it, but given how they think about Africa, I said no. I am more conscious of my Blackness and more proud of it.

Joy is a 22-year-old Zimbabwean woman from a large and close-knit family that encouraged her to be proud of her country but also to be aware of its shortcomings. She is studying health sciences in southern China. In her comments, she illustrates one way of managing the ambivalent ascriptions of Blackness by taking a nuanced and expansive view:

> Sometimes I think it [Blackness] is a curse. I am very straightforward, so I don't make anyone make me feel inferior. As a (part-time language) teacher, it is hard as they do not think that any Africans speak English. You must have confidence, you must fight. I am not defeatist. They are fascinated by us, they want to be around me, and sometimes, they are scared. Here you stop being a Zimbabwean, you are an African.

Dezite is a 36-year-old Beninese man who runs a trading business between China and West Africa. Prior to coming to Guangzhou 5 years ago, he was a trader in West Africa. He takes a more dystopian perspective when he remarks that "in Africa we do not love each other. If we did we would not come to another country. Some Blacks will treat you well; others will steal your mother."

Then there are those whose ancestors came from Africa and who incorporate that lineage into their national and ethnic identity. Such national (such as British), regional (such as West Indian), and ethnic (such as African American) identifications can privilege the link to Africa or coexist with it. One can find such Africana persons from the Americas, the Caribbean, and various European countries residing in China.

William is a 35-year-old designer from the Bahamas who has been in Shanghai for 4 years. Prior to that, he worked for extensive periods of time both in the United States and Taiwan, where a peer recruited him to work in China. He anchors his positive sense of being Black to his very being:

> [Blackness] is not a color; it is a very profound understanding of where I came from ... who I am beneath the pigment as a spiritual soul. What I bring to the world as being part of this powerful race of people. I have never been so in love with my Blackness. I didn't understand it back in the Bahamas.

Thomas, who is a 39-year-old man of West African and French heritage, has been working in Hong Kong and Shanghai for the past 12 years. He has worked in a variety of positions, including being an entertainment executive, and a marketing manager; currently, he is the chief executive director of a design boutique. He draws on his early attachments and experiences of socialization to validate his positive sense of Blackness: "What my mother gave us was a sense of belonging. We never questioned whether we were Black or White. Blackness was not negotiable. My mother was White." Such an inclusive upbringing, however, also included for Thomas the experience of being an outsider and learning to manage the challenges that often come with such a position: "Coming from a bi-cultural background, I was not locked into France. In France I was a foreigner so it did not bother me."

Chinese Ascriptions

The second commonality for conceptualizing Blackness in China deals with the varied ascriptions placed on Africana individuals by diverse elements of Chinese culture. Africana people must be cognizant of these projections, as they influence how many Chinese persons perceive them; these projections can also influence how Africana persons respond.

Garba is a 35-year-old Malian man who has been working in Shanghai for the past 10 years, most recently as a senior administrator at an international high school. Prior to that job, he worked as a sales person in financial services after a long stint teaching English as a Second Language in small southern Chinese cities. These experiences have resulted in him beginning to appreciate the positive features of Africa over time. He states:

> The Chinese value wealth beyond reason; there is no morality. It makes me think a lot about how different Africa is. I just wanted to leave Africa but now I want a more positive perception of Africa. I see myself as a change agent. How I conduct myself influences how Africa is seen. I am more sensitive to being an African.

Renee is a 32-year-old African American woman who has been in Shanghai for the past 2 years working as a content developer for an education consortium. Prior to coming to China, she worked as a teacher in Atlanta in both public and private schools, gaining exposure to a culturally diverse student body. As part of her current job, she travels extensively in Asia. Renee feels empowered by her Blackness, remarking that "the Chinese look at me a lot and so I am more aware that I am different." She noted that when she started working with Chinese peers, she apparently was the first Africana person they had had close contact with and that she was treated "like a superstar." She continued: "In China [your Blackness] it is up front, in your face all the time. You feel unique, special. I appreciate my Blackness more. I understand better the Black diaspora. I spend time educating my roommate and other Chinese people about Blackness."

Oppression and Blackness

Especially pronounced among Africana persons who are embedded as subordinate and sometimes minority groups in the West is a shared history of being oppressed along with a resistance to that oppression. This history, driven by European colonialism and slavery, constructed Blackness as representing disavowed aspects of the human condition with "the emphasis on branding them with defining features diametrically opposed to those of the self-proclaimed standard, namely, idolatry, ignorance, ugliness, evil, treachery, savagery, and social chaos" (Torres-Saillant, 2009, p. 10). Such a construction attempts to place the Black individual outside of both humanity and civilization. Such dehumanization was necessary to justify the subjugation required to appropriate their economic surplus and to limit their political hegemony. Equally important was the integration of such a disparaging view of Blackness into the colonial epistemologies that guided education and governance in the large swath of territories controlled by the Europeans from the seventeenth to the mid-twentieth centuries (Fanon, 1967; Khanna, 2003; Wright, 2004). These negative projections were part and parcel of the epistemology of the *other*, the idea that Euro Americans projected into the social unconscious of the places they occupied, including China (Dikotter, 1992).

Many of the subjects I spoke with had experienced such discrimination in their everyday lives in China. Jay's early experiences in China offer a flavor of this inferior way of thinking about Africana persons:

> It was like you were coming from Mars. They would run away or touch you. It was very strange. I could not understand this. All the students in my class were foreign, so I did not interact much with the Chinese. One day, I wanted to get my guitar fixed. I went to a store, and everyone ran out leaving the store empty. To be a called an African was an insult. They referred you us as Hei Gui, Black devil. I had to do a lot of educating. Not many Chinese could be engaged.

And yet, it would be important to acknowledge the heterogeneity of Chinese perceptions of Africana persons in China, as one also typically hears these responses, as is made clear by comments such as these from Cecilia:

> It depends on which Chinese people you are with. Sometimes I am like a celebrity; drinks, pictures. When I went to a Chinese village, they all came out, invited me to their homes. [They would engage in] dialogue. Sometimes you meet the haters. Negative vibes. Seventy percent of them are good.

In addition, there is also a widespread perception among Africana persons that money trumps race: According to Cibana, "They do not focus on you if you are Black or White, but how much money you have."

Eurocentric Construction of Blackness and Its Limitations

When combined with an ethically challenged Eurocentric exceptionalism (Powell, 1965; Somerville et al., 2009), which made them disingenuous arbiters of who was outside the pale of the civilized world, Africana persons were not only silenced, but also displaced and exploited. Such silencing speaks to a willful denial of the richness of their subjectivities and limits an acknowledgement of them to a negatively inscribed exteriority (Coates, 2015; Gordon, 2000). The Black body and mind became a container for the disavowed primitivity and inhumanity of the Eurocentric psyche; at the same time, this globally disseminated Eurocentrism denied the basic humanity and accompanying entitlements of Black people.

John, the Nigerian trader, reflects this in his perception of the Chinese persons he has interacted with:

> Most think they are smarter than us. They will change their offers and will become rude when confronted. You cannot involve the

> authorities. The guidelines keep changing so you have to be vigilant, otherwise they will find a way to cheat you. They are surprised that we foreigners are smart.

This model reduces Africana people to their exteriority and denies their rich interiority, the validity of the life lived: "he is 'out there' without an inside" (Gordon, 2000, p. 33). And therefore Eurocentric theories would have them believe that the sum total of their interior experiences constitute a false history.

Emeline's experience reflects this emphasis by some Chinese persons on the exterior as a critical marker:

> Shade of skin color is very important. The whiter you are, the higher your status in Chinese culture. During the summer, I go to the beach and I get a tan. In the winter I am "whiter," said my Chinese friend. She said that in the winter I look very good, "Your skin is very pale, much nicer."

Given the frequent privileging of a Eurocentric perspective by elites, including some in China, from a historiographical perspective one must be wary of the assumptions that Western historians make including how they have defined Africa at various points in the past. This would include the artificial limits that they have placed on what Africans can or cannot do (Keita, 2005). It was noted, for example, that many Western historians take as a given that the Indian Ocean was a barrier to trade and cultural exchange between Africa and Asia, while others have shown this to not be the case, revealing rich historical links between Africa and China (Keita, 2005). Such revelations would suggest that issues of the historical presence of Blacks in China, among other places, are under-thematized. Picking up on this theme, Keita (2005) bemoans the lack of intellectual suppleness in recognizing and examining the myriad ways in which Blackness contributes to overlap and hybridities that transcend national boundaries.

The attempts by European elites to present themselves as superior and to perceive other racial and ethnic groups as inferior were psychologically costly for the subordinated groups. Fanon (1967) was one of the first to explore the effects of the marginalization of the subjective world on the quality of the psychic life of colonial subjects. He argues that the interest in the Black is limited to his or her capacity to work, with no corresponding interest in his or her subjectivities (Gordon, 2000). This resonates with the experience of some Africana technocrats in Shanghai, who felt that some of their Chinese peers were only interested in their technical skill sets.

Some of the Africana persons I spoke to in China reflected that this narrow sense of the Black self, had its origins in their respective home countries. Such places, given their respective legacies of oppression, oftentimes limited ontological reflections and possibilities for personal growth. It is interesting to note the overlap in sentiments between those Africana persons whose home culture was a former colony and those whose home was the former colonial overlord.

Thomas, who grew up in France, made this observation with regard to constraints on his development:

> I was tired of racism; not going forward. I was about to graduate and [had] one exam to go. One of the top professors said to me, "You will have to work like a nigger slave." He was shocked when others looked at him, but he never apologized. I left and never went back. My aunt said, "Don't worry." I am a fighter of injustice; could not accept it.

Bill, an African American man from California, portrays the limits on him as follows:

> Home in the [United] States was a learning experience; it prepared me for life. When I was running my construction business, I would sound White on the phone, but when I turned up, and they saw I was Black the client's expression would change. Dignity and intelligence is put into question on a daily basis. It made me a better person. In China, they think of you as an American first not Black first.

These experiences speak to Fanon's observation that the Black person is keenly aware that he or she is often perceived through a "White gaze" with its attendant negative ascriptions (Hook & Truscott, 2013). Africana individuals are aware of this negative perception of themselves, and it will influence how they act. Many of the subjects, especially those who spoke Chinese, would report being referred to in derogatory ways. Others reported being refused job interviews and being told that the prospective employer was looking for a White person.

In this context, Frosh's (2013) observation is useful—that the social unconscious does carry racist aspects that in turn influence how the individual constructs race. Racist projections emanating from the socializing institutions and narratives of the dominant culture unconsciously inform how a given individual thinks about race and those deemed to be other. Frosh argues that we tend to not appreciate how these social projections influence intrapsychic functioning.

Blackness as Being Human

Despite the history of dehumanizing those who are of Africana heritage, one paradoxical effect has been to affirm the humanity of such persons. Cannon (in Howe, 2006) writes as much: "Black life is more than defensive reactions to oppressive circumstances of anguish and desperation. Black life is the rich, colorful creativity that emerged and reemerges in the Black quest for human dignity" (p. 425). For many Africana persons, there is an obligation to pursue ethical ways of achieving such dignity.

Freire (2000) has noted that a fundamental paradox of oppression is that such subjugation can make oppressed people aware of what aspect of their humanity it is that the oppressor wishes to subdue. Such reflection can then fuel resistance and encourage attempts to express one's humanity. So, while the Africana person is often a target of oppression, there is often resistance to such oppression. Such resistance would show itself in many ways, such as investing in a beauty salon that catered to the needs of Black women. Another form of resistance is mobilizing for immigration and justice rights as the Africans in Guangzhou have done.

Jay noted, "[I am] Still proud. What I faced made me like being Black. [It] Strengthened my position with being Black; made me proud. I had to be blacker than Black. Made me like my country more." He spoke to working in different Asian cultures representing Chinese investors and having to be resilient in the face of their skepticism about his competencies. They eventually realized that he was very good at his work.

Such affirmation is a necessary response to attempts to dehumanize persons of Africana heritage. Especially among the low-income traders in southern China, life can be hellish (Haugen & Diederich, 2016). In Guangzhou, they must be vigilant and assertive, as the immigration authorities target Blacks, assuming they are all in the country with lapsed visas engaging in illegal activities.

Africana people in China must deal with the issue of exclusion based on language, culture of origin, and physical appearance in a world where they yearn to be accepted; yet they often find themselves constructed as a problem. Most Africana persons in China do not speak the language and therefore found it difficult to develop close relationships with the Chinese. Some who do report difficulty developing substantive relationships. Yet there were others with effort developed such relationships facilitated by their efforts to acquire Chinese language skills. Given the complexity of this issue—a complexity that includes motivations, language proficiency, relational desires, and persistence, it would be rash to assert an implacable resistance on the part of the Chinese to understand Africana persons.

By paying attention to "the creases within Blackness" (Torres-Saillant, 2009, p. 19), one leaves open the possibility of new ways of thinking (Scott, 2005). So, while this holds open the possibility of revision, it also suggests that there is always the risk of regression and failure. Hence migration should be thought of as a way of working on life projects, self-discovery, and fulfillment. In a culture where there is active encouragement to exercise agency in relation to the market, there is the risk of developing self-projects with a focus on the material to the detriment of the emotional and the spiritual. So, there is the familiar neoliberal penalty of having materials but feeling emotionally impoverished. Others are not even able to accumulate wealth given the challenges of adapting to what initially appears to be a racist culture. Such individuals often leave China embittered.

Renee, the African American publishing executive, notes:

> I am more spiritually aware. I go to Buddhist retreats. I am now able to cope with how people make you feel as a Black person in China. Two to three hundred days of people staring at you; no exposure to Blacks. Something you must put up with. So after 1 year, I am a different person. I have a higher level of confidence. I had the courage to come here and I am doing well. I needed people more when I came here. I am now more self-sufficient; more of a problem solver. I do a lot of stuff on my own.

Challenge of Blackness

Given the multiplicity of ways in which Africana individuals define their Blackness, including avoidance, it is often defined on a boundary. This is the point that defines the individual in contrast to what is on the other side of the boundary; it is where difference becomes evident. This difference need not be material; as such racialized self-definitions can be a way of satisfying an existential need to belong given the decline in kinship and community bonds. Such a relationship does not require a tight link to an ethnic or racial group, as one's identity can also be defined at the boundary between self and myriad groupings (Chun, 2009).

There is a subset of Africana persons in China who felt no need for Africana group support. Renee was very clear on this issue, stating that "I do not rely on support groups. I am very self-sufficient. I pull away from group support. I am not here wishing I was home and feeling sad and lonely." While she draws on her rich cultural experiences as an African American, she feels no need for regular group validation. By way of illustration, Naujoks (2010) argues that one can identify with aspects of African culture but not necessarily identify with Africa and certainly not consider oneself African. Therefore, some forms of identification are not necessarily tightly linked to a specific racial, ethnic or national group but could be linked to a nation-based or regionally based diaspora.

Cibana exemplifies this when he notes:

> You must have an open mind as life is short. You must be vigilant regarding those who use religion or race to limit possibilities.

> Blacks who use skin color as excuses. They focus on limits, not on possibilities. Be aware of the value you add. Do not be defensive. Do a lot of educational work about Blackness. Speak to strengths. I will forget at a conference that I am the only Black and I will present in Chinese. I am unique; it is magic. Create a positive way. In a global world you cannot emphasize Blackness.

Hall (1990) notes that given a non-essentialist approach to constructing Blackness, there are myriad ways in which it can be defined. One important consequence of this approach is that there is no universally accepted way of constructing the relationship between the person of Africana heritage and Africa. So, for many in the African diaspora—those born and socialized outside of the continent—Africa remains a mythical place constructed to suit their ontological needs and the epistemological needs of the groups they are embedded in. Many of these people of Africana heritage belong to diasporas informed by African traditions, but not exclusively so. For others, Africa is imagined as disaggregated and is not necessarily conceptualized as an orienting whole. Raoul's perspective reflects one of many ways of being Black that stresses both his pride in being Black and him grounding himself as an ethical human being:

> I am a more world-wide Black person than just a Black. ... Do not do a typical Blackness but understand difference, most important is not how Black but are you a good Black. Demonstrate to others that we can be embraced like others in the world.

Hall (1990), in speaking of Blacks in the diaspora, notes the importance of recognizing the diversity within Blackness as a reinforcement of his point that there is no such thing as a pure Blackness:

> The diaspora experience as I intend it here is defined not by essence or purity, but by the recognition of a necessary heterogeneity and diversity; by a conception of identity, which lives with and through, not despite difference; by hybridity. Diaspora identities are those which are constantly producing and reproducing themselves anew, through transformation and difference.
>
> (p. 235)

Cibana, the business consultant, speaks to the differences within diverse and changing constructions of Blackness when he notes:

> We have an association of Africans who have been here for more than 10 years. We socialize together every 2 or 3 months. There are a lot of intercultural marriages. These get-togethers allow

> our children to socialize with each other. There are differences with new world Blacks. They distance from us, they stick with their own community. … It is not that they do not like us. It is not the color, it is the culture. If they think there are benefits and commonalities. … Even Africans are not together because we are Africans.

So, while there may be a good common working positive, albeit fragile, ethnic group identity by the in-group as an act of solidarity, such a commonality as a group sits alongside diverse individual definitions of ethnic identity that are rarely homogeneous, despite the tendency of out-groups to perceive it that way. An enlightened sense of Blackness would therefore speak to heterogeneity rather than some elusive essence.

One consequence of accepting Black heterogeneity is accepting that there are Africana persons who act in unethical ways but are still part of the Black mosaic (Okpewho, 2009). Emma, the prominent Nigerian community leader in Guangzhou, speaks to this diversity and the policing of the unethical:

> We also try to stop Nigerians coming in to commit crimes. We created a team called Peacekeepers, to stop these people who were making problems for everyone. Whatever the Chinese apply to the Nigerians who are behaving badly they apply to all Black people as they think all Black people are Nigerians, as we are the largest group of Africans, so any crime that is committed, they blame the Nigerians. So we arranged the Peacekeepers: Every country would have 10 people who could talk to the Chinese authorities. They would also police their communities, and try to work out problems within the community. We do not deal with serious crimes. We try to get rid of the bad elements in the community as it tarnishes everyone's reputation. We have to keep our house in order.

Inherent in being a member of a minority community is the demand for representation: the necessity of being a good ambassador for one's group. This was a recurrent theme among many Africana persons in China. Melinda's observations about the demands of Blackness were pretty typical:

> There has not been much change in how I think about my Blackness. I am pretty much the same. I am not as proud or strong. There is a lot of negativity regarding Black Americans on television. So, in someone ways I have to prove myself, be on my best behavior. I do not need to be as strong here as in America. [My Blackness] is more pronounced in the States.

Natasha, like other African Americans in China, linked the idea of representation to her experiences in the United States dealing with a majority White culture when she said that:

> I more see it as I need to show the Chinese that Black people are everywhere, not just in Africa. I feel more contented as I see the Chinese do the [skin-] whitening thing. It reminds what we Black folks go through with our color complex; you have to be proud and show a positive image. You must be the best as you must deal with White people and their racism; must be almost a perfect person showing a good reputation.

Social Support and Blackness

Africana support groups in China serve as a safe space within which to have commonalities around being an Africana person validated. Consistent theoretically with Critical Race Theory (Crenshaw et al., 1995), such groups facilitate the expression of diverse epistemologies that constitute Blackness by avoiding essentializing and homogenizing tendencies and instead promoting the recognition and appreciating of diversity within some shared commonalities around Blackness. With the goal of constructing a meaningful sense of Blackness as one of the ongoing developmental tasks of the groups, such spaces also help bring into focus unique ways of resisting oppressive, hegemonic, and often racist epistemologies and the policies and procedures they give rise to. Such support also allows for the acknowledgement of Africana diversity—work that can be done with the recognition of the uniqueness of the self. Finally, these spaces allow for understanding the constraints on being an Africana person in China and the strategies for adaptively managing the ambivalences that arise.

Harry, the French-Malian financial services executive, speaks to the importance of the group for socializing Africana persons into adaptive ways of being in China:

> We are all away from family. … Black community is trying to be as tight as possible. … We all come from different countries trying to find something new. So we all want something different, not the same but the Black community helps us to adjust here. How you present yourself is important (for) your reputation. It is a jungle out there and they are surprised when they see Blacks, Chinese, and foreigners working together.

Dean speaks to the support derived from the Caribbean Association in China (CAC) that is based in Shanghai, "The CAC makes me feel I am part of something bigger than me. When I am lonely, [it] gives me a sense of belonging. We act as brother and sister, we encourage each other."

Self and Blackness

Africana persons in China are unique individuals, and while they are constituted in part by shared cultural commonalities, they cannot be reduced to them. I heard consistently that being in China allowed Africana people to more fully experience their subjectivities around being individuated; they did not feel that they were simply reduced to being Black. In that sense, China provided the opportunity to sculpt a model of Blackness that, in part, meets their developmental needs. I am arguing here that Africana people are working on developing and understanding themselves, and that happens at times, but not always, from the perspective of being an Africana person in China. Their developmental need to be skilled, to relate well, and to increase their sense of agency is informed by their Blackness but cannot be reduced to that. In China, they may be sensitive to how their ethnicity and Chinese ascriptions with regard to Blackness impact self-work. This allows the individual to appreciate both commonalities and differences with peers, to develop an awareness of the multiple factors that over-determine what it means to be a person of Africana heritage (Cross & Fhagen-Smith, 2001).

Those factors would include the reality of social resistance as reflected in Ademoyo (2009) skepticism of Hall's position of an unfettered space within which to construct one's own subjective sense of being an Africana-informed person. Ademoyo argues instead that while an Africana-themed heritage acts as a buffer against the dehumanizing effects of slavery and colonialism, there are conditions within contemporary cultures that place restrictions on such self-work. Echeruo (1999) speaks to this ontological constraint when he notes that the Africana person has less room to maneuver than he thinks and that our history of being Black, and that of the groups such persons are embedded in, will always inform how one does the subjective work of being Black.

Jamaica Kincaid (1983), notes that there are myriad ways in which Blackness becomes a part of the individual. Blackness comes unbidden to the Africana individual and represents a lifelong ontological struggle to embrace, distance, accept, and perhaps transcend as a fundamental aspect of being. Sometimes, she speaks to the coexistence of both intimacy and distance implied in Blackness; in other settings, Kincaid addresses the rage that this understanding engenders in her, given the predations of the English that led to complex and sometimes negatively tinged ways of being Black. What is especially illuminating is her articulation of the varied aspects of Blackness that she carries and both the silencing and validation that can co-occur. Implied in this particular rendering of the term, as well as the lived experience of it, is the potential of other forms of Blackness that up until now have been obscured and that await discovery and development. Ambivalence and adaptive ways of managing such a stance toward one's Blackness is therefore an inherent feature of the self-defining and improving work of the Africana person.

Marie's experiences capture this sense of the complexity and over-determined sense of being an Africana person in China. She is a 31-year-old African American woman who is studying Chinese and who has also been working in China for 3 years. Previously, she had worked for many years as an operations manager at various electronics companies. She had previously visited China twice, and she observed that her family traveled a lot and enrolled her and her brother in a diverse set of cultural activities. She maintained diverse friendships.

Marie grew up for the most part in a suburban White neighborhood in California with very few African Americans and had to deal with being perceived as different:

> I started there in the fourth grade, and there were five other Black kids in the entire school. The White kids would touch my hair when my mom straightened it. In middle school, where there were more Black kids they called me "Oreo." [An Oreo is a biscuit sandwich that is white on the inside and black on the outside.] I was also a jock, and into science and each group would not know who I was today.

Going to a traditional Black college, she was again perceived by her peers as different, as not quite fitting into their notion of Blackness: "I fit into my own role and spent a lot of time educating people as to how I was different, that although I did not fit the ghetto stereotype I was not born with a silver spoon in my mouth."

Following intense language classes, Marie is now literate and fluent in Chinese. Her pathway was atypical as she engaged an elderly Chinese man to tutor her:

> I call him "Grandpa." He started by tutoring me, and then we became friends. If I was sick he would come with medicine and soup as he knows I like soup. He treats me as if I am one of his children; checks up on me. When my parents came to visit, he showed them around when I was at work.

At the same time, she has jarring encounters that remind her that she is not Chinese:

> I am always educating people. When they say something to me in Chinese, I respond in Chinese. They will insist that I am still not one of them. This is a legacy you have as an African American

> that is the kind of treatment you get in the States and it toughens your skin for when you go overseas.

Marie perceives her experiences around being different as having made her stronger:

> I love being an African American Black. When there are racist occurrences, the fact that I am me and can teach other people; I can teach Caucasians how to deal with racism as I have had to deal with it. I am a bridge; I do not feel that I am being pushed down.

Blackness is initially inscribed on individuals, and many spend a lifetime seeking to make sense of it, limiting the effects of its negative ascriptions, and exploiting its links to innovation and love, while ideally incorporating it into fulfilling and productive ways of being in the world.

I approached the meaning of Blackness in China cautiously, as my travel experiences and readings made me aware that there was no universal cultural algorithm that enabled one to quickly understand racial and ethnic hierarchies in a given culture. I am always sensitive of my Blackness when being in predominantly non-Black spaces and when encountering non-Africana persons.

Occasionally, while in China I would see a person of obvious Africana lineage. Some of the Africana persons would acknowledge me, and some looked straight through me. Initially, I found the lack of response bewildering. It took me many years of traveling in Asia to figure out that my New World experience of Blackness especially in Canada and the United States, where to be Black is perceived as different, meant that we were apt to acknowledge each other as compatriots when in non-Black spaces. This however was simply not a dynamic that occurred regularly in Asia. For many Africana persons from Africa, the key marker of commonality was not visible Blackness, but ethnic and national signifiers; there is no history for many of them of a commonality based on merely being dark-skinned. I wondered, given that Africana persons in China are clearly a minority and are perceived as a homogeneous group, if a sense of Africana commonality would evolve, akin to what one observes in the United States and Canada.

The Africana person's experience in China is varied, but with this unrepresentative sample, arcs toward being positive. There is a stated need for unblinking vigilance given the ever-present necessity to compete for resources in a cultural space that can be quite biased toward the foreigner. The self-management needs are complex and emotionally costly, but there is a sense that a sojourn in China can be intellectually and materially profitable, if emotionally bracing. Africana persons who do well in China have learned to adaptively manage the mixed feelings generated by the realities of China. They have also developed an appreciation that to some degree home needs to be portable, while other aspects must be mourned given their unattainability.

References

Ademoyo, A. (2009). The ontological imperative for the new African diaspora. In I. Okpewho & N. Nzegwu (Eds.), *The new African diaspora* (pp. 501–518). Bloomington, IN: Indiana University Press.

Asante, M. (1993). Racism, consciousness and Afrocentricity. In G. Early (Ed.), *Lure and loathing: Essays on race, identity, and the ambivalence of assimilation* (pp. 127–143). New York, NY: Penguin.

Chun, A. (2009). On the geopolitics of identity. *Anthropological Theory*, *9*(3), 331–349.

Coates, T. (2015). *Between the world and me*. New York, NY: Spiegel & Grau.

Crenshaw, K., Gotanda, N., Peller, G., & Thomas, K. (Eds.). (1995). *Critical race theory: The key writings that informed the movement*. New York, NY: The New Press.

Cross, W., & Fhagen-Smith, P. (2001). Patterns of African-American Identity Development: A Life-Span Perspective. In C. L Wijeyesinghe & B. W Jackson (Eds.), *New perspectives on racial identity development: A theoretical and practical anthology* (pp. 243–270). New York, NY: New York University Press.

Dikotter, F. (1992). *The discourse of race in modern China*. London, UK: Hurst & Company.

Echeruo, M. (1999). An African diaspora: The ontological project. In I. Okpewho, C. Davies, & A. Mazrui (Eds.), *The African diaspora* (pp. 3–18). Bloomington, IN: Indiana University Press.

Fanon, F. (1967). *Black skin, white masks*. New York, NY: Grove Press.

Freire, P. (2000). *Pedagogy of the oppressed*. New York, NY: Continuum.

Frosh, S. (2013). Psychoanalysis, colonialism, racism. *Journal of Theoretical and Philosophical Psychology*, *33*(3), 141–154.

Gordon, L. (2000). *Existentia Africana: Understanding Africana existential thought*. New York, NY: Routledge.

Hall, S. (1990). Cultural identity and diaspora. In J. Rutherford (Ed.), *Identity, community, culture and difference* (pp. 222–237). London, UK: Lawrence & Wishart.

Haugen, H., & Diederich, M. (2016). Life in China. Retrieved from https://uturnasia.com/2016/01/24/test-1/

Hook, D., & Truscott, R. (2013). Fanonian ambivalence: On psychoanalysis and postcolonial critique. *Journal of Theoretical and Philosophical Psychology*, *33*(3), 155–169.

Howe, L. (2006). Enchantment, weak ontologies and administrative ethics. *Administration & Society*, *38*(4), 422–446.

Keita, M. (2005). Africans and Asians: Historiography and the long view of global interaction. *Journal of World History*, *16*(1), 1–30.

Khanna, R. (2003). *Dark continents: Psychoanalysis and colonialism*. Durham, NC: Duke University Press.

Kincaid, J. (1983). *At the bottom of the river*. New York, NY: Farrar Straus Giroux.

Naujoks, D. (2010). Diasporic identities: Reflections on transnational belongings. *Diaspora Studies*, *3*(1), 1–21.

Okpewho, I. (2009). Introduction: Can we go home again? In I. Okpewho & N. Nzegwu (Eds.), *The new African diaspora* (pp. 3–30). Bloomington, IN: Indiana University Press.

Powell, E. (1965). Speech at Wolverhampton. Retrieved from www.enochpowell.net/fr81.html

Scott, D. (2005). Stuart Hall's ethics. *Small Axe*, *17*(9), 1–16.

Somerville, W., Sriskandarajah, D., & Latorre, M. (2009). United Kingdom: A reluctant country of immigration. *Migration Policy Institute*. Retrieved from www.migrationpolicy.org/article/united-kingdom-reluctant-country-immigration

Torres-Saillant, S. (2009). One and divisible: Mediations on global Blackness. *Small Axe*, *29*(13), 4–25.

Wright, M. (2004). *Becoming Black: Creating identity in the African diaspora*. Durham, NC: Duke University Press.

8 Conclusions and Possibilities for the Future

Africana workers, while profiting from being in China, struggle to have their socio-emotional needs met, and they must therefore not be too invested in staying there. They must adaptively manage the ambivalence that comes with living in in-tween spaces, no matter where they reside.

The presence of a slowly growing cohort of Afro-Chinese families, the demands of a globalized market and the restlessness of its middle class are in tension with China's antipathy to cultural difference and unscripted social change. For the foreseeable future it is difficult to make any predictions about the viability of doing Africana identity work in China

China's ongoing modernization program offers both opportunity and limitations to the skilled Africana worker. In addition to their earnings there is the opportunity to work on self-development projects around issues such as identity, increasing knowledge about self in the world, and more nuanced and robust ways of being reflective. Structural conditions in China can make it challenging to do such self-work. While China actively seeks out skilled foreigners, including Africana workers, it still strives to achieve its goal of ensuring that China remains a culturally homogeneous society. It is not clear how China will manage its antipathy toward the foreigner and yet be an integral member of a culturally diverse international community and economic system. The long-term outcome for Africana workers in China hinges on continued demand for their skills and the evolution of human rights in China.

The Challenges

Managing Uncertainty

The modern individual exists in a world rife with uncertainty. The environment, the economy, ideologies, and ontologies are all in flux, and they appear to be highly contingent on each other, with policies, individual agency, and economic activities each influencing and being influenced by the other. The Africana person leaves home because of its suffocating policies and is drawn to China given its dynamic economy and the possibilities that offers for self-growth.

Within this turbulence, individuals yearn to be free and are emboldened by some globalized ideologies, such as liberalism, that speak to agency, autonomy, and dignity. They are able to enhance their intellectual skills, be productive, and be respected as creative and valued members of the community. For many, dignity comes from a sense of recognition of their individuality as ethnic, racial, and gendered persons. It is not limited to them being productive, although that is a component of how they assess self-growth.

Due to the insufficiency of resources at home, many venture abroad, leaving a place with a long history of community or national underdevelopment and the contemporary inequities flowing from widely adopted neoliberal policies. Such policies often produce socioeconomic arrangements that make it difficult to acquire an education at reasonable cost, and that in turn stifles the creation of high-value productivity. Thus the possibility of the individual attaining meaningful and well-paying work is reduced.

Such policies also often restrict the space for a model of self-development that aspires to more than wealth accumulation, and even for such narrow aspirations, they can make it difficult to acquire the necessary resources to develop the capabilities demanded by the market. Wherever modern individuals are located, they are confronted with the need to devote more resources to ensure that market forces do not reduce their agency to that of being consumers whose productive efforts are only in the service of them being consumers. For many individuals, it would seem that agency in the service of authenticity, accountability, and community is increasingly constrained.

Containing Ambivalence

To achieve their desired outcomes, the individual, in this case the Africana person in China finds a range of opportunities alongside substantial restraints. Such opportunities are often in the service of knowledge acquisition or present themselves as offerings tied to market-driven demands for technical skills. By contrast, the restraints are usually in areas where there are attempts to exercise agency toward challenging the political or where individuals are demanding recognition as valued members of the community. This speaks to ambivalence on the part of the host country that in turn exacerbates the foreign worker's own ambivalence. That ambivalence is fed by the psychological reality that Africana workers in China do not experience themselves as being fully fledged members of the community, but neither are those communities completely hostile to them.

This ambivalence, if adaptively managed, leaves the individual in a state of psychological in-between-ness, with a limited sense of belonging in either home or host country. This state reflects to some degree the increased ambivalence of host countries that desire the foreign workers' labor and technical skills but deny them the possibility of becoming permanent and entitled members of the host community. It also reflects a realization on the part of the individual that love for home is informed, in part, by melancholy arising from its inability to satisfy developmental needs, hence the need to leave.

The Chinese Conundrum

The situation of Africana persons in China must be seen in the context of economic, social, and political factors that influence their self-development but at the same time place limits on some aspects of that project. The first of these is China's rapid economic growth over the past 30 years that has moved millions of its citizens out of poverty and created a substantial middle class, allowing China to become a major producer of inexpensive goods and fueling a demand for creative workers.

These economic changes have proven attractive and beneficial to some classes of Africana foreign workers, such as transnational traders and technocrats. Given access to well-resourced nationally and regionally constituted transnational networks, many Africana workers argue that the economic benefits that, in part, drive the decision to leave home, are more attractive in China than in other possible destinations, such as Europe or the United States. This, many of them note, includes allowing for the cost of racism and other unattractive aspects of being in China.

These economic changes present both opportunities and challenges for China and by extension for Africana persons working there. The first challenge is the global nature of information and production flow, and the commodification, cost reductions, and lowering of the barriers to entry that flow from that. As China's workforce ages and wages rise, it is no longer as profitable for China to focus on low-value production, which it was more able to do when it had an abundant and inexpensive labor supply. Such production at lower cost is shifting to countries like Vietnam. As a consequence, China will increasingly focus on the production of high-value goods and services that are more profitable and that meet the raising consumerist aspirations and service demands of its growing middle class and urban population.

Such policies do not resolve a more substantive dilemma for China. Its wish for harmony within a relatively homogeneous Han-dominated society is at serious odds with the diversity strivings of some of its own minority groups. It is also at odds with China's need for the healthy infusion of diverse perspectives that provide essential fuel for the innovative practices necessary to compete in global markets. The emphasis on recreating a mythical, harmonious, and homogeneous society is in tension with the dynamic cultural diversity that neoliberalism unwittingly rewards.

There is a more subtle challenge evident in the bounded nature of agency in China; there is much latitude in relation to the market but many constraints with regard to rights demands such as adherence to rule of law, accountability, and fairness. While this is a major concern for many Africana workers in China, their miniscule numbers and outsider status do not give them much leverage. China's growing middle class is deploying such leverage, and while it is too early to say, the increase of the urban population as a strategy to increase consumer demand has implications for increased rights demands. Such demands might well improve the rights accorded to foreigners, including Africana persons who are valued for creative and innovative input. Representations by their respective governments, especially in countries where China has substantial economic and political interests, comprise an additional potential leverage point for Africana persons. From time to time, Nigeria has flexed its muscles in this regard, but that so far appears to be the exception rather than the rule. In summary, the future prospects for Africana workers in China are inseparable from human rights development, economic policy and the gyrations of the global economy.

Some Implications for Africana Workers in China

These challenges have many implications for Africana workers in China, a few of which will be mentioned here. China will cease to be attractive as a source of cheap goods, and some Africana traders will move away from China to cheaper sources, such as Vietnam. There is some anecdotal evidence that this has already begun to happen. There is also some evidence that some Africana businesspersons in Guangzhou and Yiwu have begun to invest in producing middle-to-high value goods to take advantage of increased demand in those areas. To provide such goods and services, China will continue to sharpen its focus on enticing innovative workers to come to China with attractive visa regimes and other benefits, and this is especially evident in the Africana community in Shanghai that is dominated by such technocrats. At the same time, China will continue to discourage the presence of necessity entrepreneurs and others members of the precariat. These individuals who often lack the skills and the necessary social supports to adequately address their socioeconomic needs, especially in Guangzhou, are increasingly subject to aggressive strict visa enforcement, and imprisonment, fines, and deportation.

Self and Identity Challenges for the Africana Person in China

Within this mix of contingent social forces, individuals must chart a course that will reflect their influence as an expression of substantive agency. Central to this task is the human need for recognition and positive validation as an individual and as a member of a variety of social groups. An important challenge for Africana persons in China is managing the ascription of being an ambivalently perceived *other*. This is the standard wariness of the stranger informed by China's history of foreign exploitation and its negative secondhand exposure to Africana persons. At the same time, there does not appear to be a deep-rooted hatred of Africana persons or the institutionalized racism and attendant discrimination that is evident in the West. Many Africana persons report a willingness by Chinese nationals to abandon a reactive prejudicial stance, to look beyond the negatively tinged ascription of *other* and engage them as individuals.

The work around understanding cultural difference presents a series of challenges for both parties. For the Chinese, with their emphasis on homogeneity and harmony, the cultural accommodating to the foreigner in general and to the Africana person specifically is ideologically challenging. There is the ever-present temptation to return to the spirit of the isolationist policies of the Ming dynasty, so as to minimize the undesired aspects of Western influence. At the same time, this is in conflict with Chinese involvement in the global community of nations, its involvement in international trade, and its need for exposure to creative ideas and innovative practices.

Africana workers often harbor negative cultural biases that they bring to China as a result of socialization in their respective home cultures and as a result of the initial negative response to them by some Chinese persons. To enjoy a more gratifying social experience in China requires them to acknowledge and manage these implicit biases. In addition, an investment in the seemingly daunting task of understanding the Chinese people and their varied perspectives is necessary. This would include them learning Chinese and socializing with Chinese nationals. To the extent that they are preoccupied with either acquiring market-oriented skills or deploying such skills, they may well live a narrow and unfulfilling life, bereft of any substantive exposure to Chinese culture and its people outside of the marketplace. In situations in which such a narrowing happens, they become unwittingly complicit in maintaining an austere outsider status.

Africana Ambivalence and Being Other

The Africana person, given the current cultural dynamics of China, is other, an outsider, but also occupies a place, however tentative, within China. Africana individuals have rights, however modest; garners benefits, however circumscribed; and feel that they have profited from being there, albeit a profit tinged with some bitterness.

Africana people in China have a parallel relationship to home, a place with a history of both elation and frustration, recognition and yet a sense of not-quite-belonging. In both places, they occupy a state of in-between-ness. Both places make claims on identity—home for its primordial attachments and China for an invigorating sense of themselves as innovative and productive. Yet neither fully assuages the sense of being embedded in a place that both recognizes their uniqueness and validates their disparate selves and identifications. This is both an exhilarating and risky psychological place to be, an emotionally-fueled journey orbiting many ideological suns.

From such an in-between space, they often have the bracing but refreshing and fecund observations of the outsider. It fuels their creativity, and it allows them to potentially see beyond superficial difference, identify deep commonalities, and engage carefully the differences that are beneficial to them. This can be exhilarating and is the spirit of *suzhi*, with its emphasis on self-improvement and the heightened status and esteem that comes with that. It requires them to adopt certain soft subjective essentialisms, such as the certainty of a paradoxically fluid definition of home. It becomes essential in that it is fixed, a point of reference that is central to keeping them oriented in an ever-changing intellectual, social, and ethical landscape. Paradoxically, since it often changes, its contradictions are not interrogated, and so despite its waxing and waning, it is a source of grounding yet not an everlasting dictate.

In such a space, provided the individual is resilient, there is no urgency to be explicitly fixed or to always resolve dichotomies, and the experienced anxiety is tolerated in the service of the pursuit of the novel and of being innovative. It heightens the reflective Africana person's awareness of the diversity of selves that constitute who she or he is, and that person becomes adept at knowing when and in what culture contexts to deploy a given aspect of the self. The sheer diversity of the experiences that Africana persons partake of broadens their sense of what constitutes the self in ways that are challenging and at times gratifying.

Such a position of in-between-ness comes at an emotional cost that if well managed energizes growth but if poorly managed leads to alienation and immobility. Given that there is no view from nowhere, there must be some fixity, however transient that point of pause may be. In that place, there is some mourning of the loss of some aspects of home, and a tight rein must be maintained on nostalgia, given its regressive pull. There is also the risk of reveling in belonging nowhere, in becoming overly attached to the identity of the much-vaunted cosmopolitan person who, in the extreme manifestation of such a position, seemingly eschews all cultural attachment. Favored by the cosmopolitan is a hyper-individuality based on fleeting relationships and hyper-mobility. This is evident in a certain class of Africana technocrats and to a lesser degree among some Africana traders. They do well materially, but some are stalked by loneliness that in turn is the product of long-standing problems around attachment and commitment. For them, the very mobility they treasure leaves them existentially adrift.

Eating Bitterness

Living in China, with its authoritarianism and its adoption of selective aspects of neoliberalism, generates constraints on the self that makes everyone experience *chiku* or the eating of bitterness. Eating bitterness was first discussed in Chapter 3, and it was evident the various ways that it informs and shapes the lives of Africana workers in China given certain conditions. The degree that bitterness is a component of the diet is informed by psychological and developmental factors as well as the choreography of permissiveness and authority in China. To do well in China, the individual must have the requisite foundational skills prior to arriving in China. Individuals who are psychologically resilient, socially adept, curious, and possess solid intellectual skills tend to hold their own in China. They invariably come from well-resourced networks that have facilitated them developing the necessary capabilities and the robust sense of agency that flows from that. The sense of immobility that some Africana individuals experience at home might be a result of systemic failures in the areas of intellect and technical skill acquisition. For others, the immobility is a result of socio-emotional deficits rising from predispositions and family-based deficits.

In addition, there is the enframing issue of the presence of systemic factors that require everyone living in a neoliberal-informed culture to eat bitterness, exacerbated in China by its authoritarian approach to matters political. There is a clear sense of the bitterness that arises from having to accept limits on political agency. There is also a sense of incompleteness that is experienced by individuals pursuing a lifestyle that is seemingly restricted to material accumulation and consumption with its related sense of status tied to market values.

The Inevitability of an Ambivalent Stance

Given the pervasive uncertainty of modern life, with its risks and opportunities combined with the absence of definitive guideposts, the modern individual lives with a constant feeling of ambivalence. With a surfeit of information, but in some cases a paucity of knowledge, the modern individual must be both wary and confident, hurrying carefully to improve the self while avoiding serious narcissistic injuries. Ambivalence, with its combination of confidence in the face of opportunity and anxiety in the face of risk, is very much a basic feature of the contemporary psyche. Africana workers must accept in the short-to-medium term that their difference as an outsider and as an Africana person is a strength that, if well deployed, can be a source of pleasure and profit.

This sits alongside a sense of being selectively excluded, and Africana individuals must therefore develop adaptive ways of managing the ambivalence engendered by these experienced positions. They might very well be quite familiar with such adaptations given their experiences at home, where they also had to thoughtfully manage their ambivalence that was engendered by a sense of being different and being constrained. They are able to understand their otherness and have some sense of how it is perceived by others from both a positive and agency-enhancing perspective and also in ways that limit the development of capabilities. Providing a sense of grounding for them is the ability to bring a tolerable degree of flexibility to the ethical decisions they make, knowing when to be tolerant and when to hold steadfast. Such adaptability in managing ambivalence is best achieved by a reflective stance within the context of caring relationships. The Africana person who is reflective, resilient, has the requisite capabilities and good-enough social supports is able to adaptively manage an ever-present sense of ambivalence.

Theoretical Implications of this Work

The first task is to attempt to meet de Haas's (2014) two conditions for a good-enough contribution to theorizing about migration. He argues that migration should be examined within the context of larger socioeconomic forces that influence migration, which in turn influences those forces. de Haas's second condition is the need to effectively manage the tension between understanding the complexities and differences generated by subjectivities and other elusive contingencies, while at the same time attempting to identify consistencies that would contribute to theory-making.

Agency Influencing Structure Over Time

Specific to this work on Africana persons in China and consistent with de Haas's challenge is the interplay between structure and agency. In Lian and Rahman's (2011) formulation, agency speaks to the capacity to leverage cultural capital, such as networks and skill sets, while structure speaks to the contexts in which the individual is embedded and their facilitatory or constraining features. This work speaks to both aspects of structure and agency, examining the psychosocial resources that the Africana person deploys in the varied structural settings in China. Under-thematized in the contemporary research is the degree to which agency can shift structure, in terms of policy, especially where there is mutual self-interest. This is evident in Yiwu, where the authorities are invested in building a transnational trade hub, and therefore are sensitive to the needs of the Africana business community there (Cisse, 2015). Given the importance of increased innovation and productivity to China's economic strategies, Africana workers who excel in such areas will continue to find China attractive. Such contributions might well give them leverage to garner greater accessibility to permanent residence status and substantive inclusion in China.

The economic power of foreign workers within the host country is often conceptualized as being limited to their consumption power, and is generally thought of as negligible in relation to their ability to affect structural arrangements. As transnational movements increase, this is a position that will have to be re-conceptualized to examine the gradual shift toward mutual interests. This is especially the case where transnational workers are in demand for their scarce and specialized technical skills. As a rule, intelligent individuals over time will not be satisfied with second-class and subordinate status. Their hopes will resonate with the much larger cohort of their equally smart and restless Chinese peers.

The Power of Capital

Such a shift would speak to Bourdieu's (Van Hear, 2014) observation of the increasingly diverse nature of capital, with an emphasis on its transformational potential. Here, I am thinking of the intellectual capital that the Africana person brings to China and the possibility of it being transformed into economic capital with its material benefits as well as cultural capital and the enhanced esteem that comes with that. Intellectual capital is in high demand and has two positive implications for Africana persons in China. There is recognition of them, along with other creative and innovative foreigners, as having capital resources that are in high demand.

This in turn influences structure as manifested in adjustments to China's visa policies in order to attract such capital. It also has the effect of generating ascriptions of esteem by the Chinese toward the talented Africana person, in contrast to the traditional negative ascriptions projected on to Africana persons. The seeming fluidity of ascriptions in the context of the discovery of capital writ large is an intriguing feature of China, and is another under-thematized area of research. It is in contrast to the dominance of the seeming solidity of the negative Euro American view of Africana people, with an accompanying underappreciation of their capital. It is possible that the imperatives of the marketplace—the relentless pursuit of novelty and profit—will temper the irrational fears that drive the negative ascribing of the Africana person. In addition, what is also not thoroughly understood are the processes by which the individual negotiates the minefield of being both desired and feared.

Subjectivity, Ambition, and Inequality

Psychoanalysis is ideally well suited to explore the complexity of the subjective, where desire, fear, irrationality, and dispassion are in ever-shifting combinations of conflict, cooperation, and compromise. It allows us to understand the dynamics of in-between-ness and the anxieties, ambivalences, and adaptations that it generates. Hope is stalked by dread, and ambition is shadowed by doubt. These are played out in the lives of those who venture out from home and are subject, to some degree, to the vicissitudes of the marketplace and their ability to act, when necessary, against its commodifying current. In an age of marked inequality and dehumanization, it is not clear how some are able to thrive despite the odds.

That being said, the traditional psychoanalytic approach to migration speaks to the trauma of loss and has little to say about the discovery of agency and the management of in-between-ness. Equally troubling, especially in American psychoanalytic thinking, is the mostly incurious stance toward the sociopolitical. Although relational models have dabbled in that area, it is most prominent in its focus on feminist themes; the other, when mentioned, is limited to intrapsychic musings. As a result, the influence of the sociopolitical, with reference to capital and race, is grossly under-thematized. Africana persons constructs embedded in racism, inequality, and the resilience that they project are theoretically underdeveloped. Also missing are thoughts about the strategies that enables them to thrive in inhospitable spaces and over time affect changes in those spaces.

So, it is difficult to appreciate the subjectivities of the Africana perspective given the limitations of a psychoanalysis of the refused *other*. Given its dystopian biases, psychoanalysis tends to emphasize the failings and vulnerabilities of the Africana person, among others, and this is the case even when, as exemplified in Fanon's work, attention is paid to the damage that a hostile culture can visit on the Africana psyche. The adaptation, as exemplified in the pioneering work of DuBois (2007), whose double consciousness speaks to ambivalence, is not a feature of psychoanalytic core thinking, even when on the rare occasion it is brought to bear on Africana ways of being in the world.

Psychoanalysis does, however, offer some possibilities. It sensitizes us to the psychological physics of time: the idea that the past is also in some ways the present, and if effectively mined allows some sculpting of the future. There is a sub-cohort of Africana persons who are adept at managing themselves from an in-between perspective, a place that offers the potential to integrate different perspectives across time and space with favorable outcomes. Their approach to self-management in a place of uncertainty is a manifestation of Mitchell's (1993) assertions of the multiple aspects of selves that we deploy in contemporary settings.

The Pleasures of Being Other

There are often unacknowledged pleasures that come with being the outsider. As a consequence of nativism, among other factors, the *othe*r can increasingly remain the *other*, but in more differentiated ways than was previously possible. There are pleasures to be derived from a position that is not unthoughtfully dependent on mindless validation of a commodified and unsurprising self. There is no inevitable desire for the death of former selves or for the holding on to obsolete perspectives and inhibitions. There is a freedom that, although sometimes costly to attain, allows for reimagining the self and can lead to recognition of aspects of the self that have been marginalized by the tyranny of unhealthy aspects of the normative.

Given that they have not completely relinquished the home country, it would be illuminating to know the psychic transformations that someone undergoes to remain in a place of gratification and not be too regressively nostalgic, nor do they have to be emphatically repudiated. By necessity, the foreigner must have a home within the mind that has both essentialized and mutable components, thereby allowing for aspects to be appropriately deployed as reassurance and as caution. Such a home speaks to the paradox of otherness: No matter how different one might be, it is within a context of commonality with others in a shared humanity. Psychoanalysis is adept at speaking to the alienation, especially among immigrants, that arises from being perceived as too different (Strenger, 2013, 2016). There is a case, made so often in psychoanalysis, about the losses that result from fleeing for literal life and the impossibility of return. For some Africana people in China, there is indeed a sense of the dark side of in-between-ness, a sense of failure at home and failure in China, and a sense of the unsuccessful attempt to flee from the self.

This work raises the possibility that some foreign workers in the host country do face challenges inherent in being outsiders. They are not, however, necessarily preoccupied with loss nor are they striving to be assimilated. Many of them are capable of managing well a sense of in-between-ness that does not require the despair of outsider-ness or the cultural surrender that comes with assimilation.

A thoughtful psychoanalysis would profit from beginning to examine its uncritical alignment with the normative. The extant psychoanalytic literature values (and only values) the seemingly mindless dynamics of adaptation, which becomes unwittingly privileged when theorists focus on assimilation to the host country as a purely positive goal, and as the only process available to people working in a country other than their home country.

Identity and the Challenges of Community

What are not as well thematized are the social supports that might facilitate the individual's strivings. Given their relatively recent arrival and the transient nature of most of the Africana population in China, it does not fit the traditional definition of a diasporic grouping. There is no large and long-established core grouping, and it does not have a strong common identity. What is common is a diverse set of identifications with Africa or African culture—itself a diverse set of constructions—and homogenizing ascriptions by the Chinese as Africans, regardless of their country or region or ethnicity of origin.

The view from the host country is traditionally a crucial factor in shaping community among the foreign population, but that tends to be more influential where the incoming groups are migrants determined to stay and establish a new home. They are therefore invested in assimilating to some degree into the new culture that in turn to some degree facilitates achieving this goal. Increasingly, many transnational workers find themselves in these transient spaces that have homelike and diasporic features but are not a transition into permanent residence or citizenship in the host country. More work has to be done on the phenomenon of long-term intermittent or almost-permanent residence in a transitional space.

These "new," diaspora-like spaces have some novel features that are adaptive to the given context. They have a virtual component, evident in the Africana communities in China. In such a setting, there is continuous use of cyberspace. Laguerre (in Dufoix, 2008) defines "virtual diaspora" as "the use of cyberspace by immigrants or descendants of an immigrant group for the purpose of participating or engaging in online interactional transactions" while stressing that no virtual diaspora can sustain itself without real contact (p. 101). This perspective is especially resonant with the physically dispersed Africana community in Shanghai; its virtual nature enhances professional networking, but there is not sufficient direct social contact to nurture socio-emotional growth or a substantive sense of community.

Georges Prevelakis (in Dufoix, 2008) refers to a class of relationships between diasporic type networks that he refers to as a "galactic organization." This features "Independent and far flung groupings bound by a language, culture and history as against law or a hierarchal relationship. This is in contrast to a dendritic organization driven by the relationship between a center and its periphery" (pp. 38–39). This is evident in China, where the communities relate to a diverse set of other communities that may or may not be in Africa, such as Jamaican communities in North America and Europe or Nigerian communities in diverse settings within and outside of Nigeria. Such diversity speaks to the increase in migration since the end of World War II, facilitated further by increased globalization. So, within the Africana communities in China, there is no strong orientation to a shared center. Each group has its own and, within some groups, multiple homelands. What is also interesting is the Africana homogenizing by China and the need to understand and accommodate that ascription by powerful elements of the host country.

This realization of a shared Blackness/Africanness is embraced by some as a validation of an aspect of their identity to which they had not previously given much thought. This creates the possibility of a sense of Africana identity that celebrates differences within a deeper if not always well understood common relationship to Africa as a cultural identity writ large and informed by its diaspora. It would also be a psychosocial necessity in China given the tendency of many Chinese persons to homogenize Blackness.

Future Possibilities

The demographics of the Africana population in China will continue to shift in tandem with the needs of the Chinese economy and the rights strivings of its growing middle class. There will be fewer opportunities for providers of services that add little value and an increase in demand for those providing intellectual and financial capital. So, the cohort of small-volume traders of low-margin consumer items will decline in size. By contrast, high-end manufacturers and technocrats will continue to be in demand.

It is questionable how influential the Africana population can be in China given its small size, its dispersion, and the high level of transience of its members, most of whom are oriented toward their home culture and in some cases to an alternate host culture in the developed West. There are two modest but fascinating exceptions, the first of which is a small group of Africana-Chinese families with bicultural children who are considered Chinese nationals and whose Africana fathers have the right to live in China. There are also tantalizing hints of Chinese men who, following a work sojourn, usually in Africa, have returned to China with Africana wives. While there are Africana-Asian children in other countries, especially Vietnam, what is different in China is that many Afro-Chinese children are embedded in intact nuclear families with varying access to the support networks of both families. One can but speculate as to the long-term effect of these children on the fiction of Chinese cultural homogeneity, especially where the emphasis is on phenotypical sameness.

Part of but not limited to this grouping are Africana persons—mostly men, but also some women in Shanghai—who wish to live on a long-term basis in China and will advocate for the right to do so. This is a challenge for China, as there are often times highly credentialed and also innovative individuals that China seeks to attract and retain to raise the amount and quality of its products and services. It is not clear given China's attraction and simultaneous wariness regarding foreigners how it will accommodate such demands over time. Complicating this dilemma is the fact that some Africana rights demands resonate with those of China's nascent but evolving middle class, which cannot be as easily dismissed, given their centrality to China's ongoing push to be a first world nation.

One could therefore argue that in-between-ness might well be a stable form of psychic organization, rather than a transient one, albeit with risks. Individuals who have a healthy history of relating and belonging, while being accepted as different, are well able to manage the demand of being not quite at home, wherever they are. There exists a subgroup of psychologically healthy migrants who enjoy the peripatetic life and the sense of being outsiders, alongside reports that others are psychologically or professionally immobilized. Clearly, in-between-ness is a complex psychological space that needs further disaggregating.

There is also the intriguing age-old tension between being reflective and acting in the world. The colonial—like the cultures from which many Africana people in China hail from—often discourages reflection given the limited agency possible in those locales. Capitalism, by way of contrast, seeks to sculpt reflection in the service of an agency focused on consumption and the search for an ever elusive sense of gratification. It warrants further exploration as to the conditions and behaviors that allow individuals to pursue and at the same time accept the limits on satisfaction.

An area that also offers research possibilities is the issue of the management of intimacy among foreigners in China. Many Africana women noted the difficulty of developing sustainable relationships given their antipathy toward Chinese men and the relative unavailability of Africana men. Emma, the Nigerian community leader in Guangzhou, spoke to some of the challenges facing African men married to Chinese women. There are suggestions of bias that need exploring especially given language and other cultural challenges. Little is known about the psychosocial contours of these various relationships.

In summary, the presence of Africana persons in China reflects the continuing evolution of globalized forces across economic, social, political, and technological domains. It influences both structure and agency and that in turn influences how globalization unfolds. Africana people have been venturing from their homes for eons, pursuing *suzhi* and also eating bitterness. Their ongoing existence and their ability to thrive for the most part speak to their capacity to adapt, albeit at a price.

References

Cisse, D. (2015). African traders in Yiwu: Their trade networks and their role in the distribution of "made in China" products in Africa. *Journal of Pan African Studies*, 7(10), 44–64.

de Haas, H. (2014). Migration theory: Quo vadis? (DEMIG project paper 24, University of Oxford: International Migration Institute).

DuBois, W. E. B. (2007). *The souls of Black folks*. New York, NY: Oxford University Press.

Dufoix, S. (2008). *Diasporas*. Berkeley, CA: University of California Press.

Lian, K., & Rahman, M. (2011). From workers to entrepreneurs: Development of Bangladeshi migrant businesses in the Republic of Korea. *International Migration*, *52*(2), 122–139.

Mitchell, S. (1993). *Hope and dread in psychoanalysis*. New York, NY: Basic Books.

Strenger, C. (2013). The new cosmopolitans: Challenges and discontents. *Psychoanalytic Psychology*, *30*(2), 264–280.

Strenger, C. (2016). *Freud's legacy in the global era*. New York, NY: Routledge.

Van Hear, N. (2014). Reconsidering migration and class. *International Migration Review*, *48*(S1), 100–121.

Index

For Product Safety Concerns and Information please contact our EU representative GPSR@taylorandfrancis.com
Taylor & Francis Verlag GmbH, Kaufingerstraße 24, 80331 München, Germany

www.ingramcontent.com/pod-product-compliance
Ingram Content Group UK Ltd.
Pitfield, Milton Keynes, MK11 3LW, UK
UKHW021959180926
475701UK00003B/108
* 9 7 8 0 3 6 7 5 8 5 0 2 0 *